THE GIFT OF AGING

Award-winning authors Marcy Cottrell Houle and Elizabeth Eckstrom have teamed up again following the success of their critically acclaimed book *The Gift of Caring*, winner of the 2016 National Christopher Award. This new book blends frontline science with inspirational stories and insights from wise elders for aging with health, joy, and purpose. The book explains how our bodies and brains age, defining what can be expected with aging and what is unusual. It demonstrates ways we can significantly increase our chances for a positive aging experience into our 80s, 90s, and 100s. It offers key strategies for meeting the challenges of aging, informs us of issues of inclusion and equity, and advises on handling legal and financial affairs. *The Gift of Aging* illustrates how we can make the third act of our lives meaningful and fulfilling, ensuring we as elders can make a difference in our world.

Marcy Cottrell Houle, MS, is a professional wildlife biologist and the author of eight award-winning books. Two of her books received the Christopher Award "for books that affirm the highest values of the human spirit." Her work has been selected by the *New York Times* as a Best Book for Earth Day. She is a contributing opinion writer for the *New York Times*, *LA Times*, and *Globe and Mail*, and has written articles for the *Nature Conservancy Magazine*, *Cricket Magazine for Children*, *Reader's Digest*, the *New York Times*, and *Smithsonian Magazine*. Marcy lives with her family on a small farm on Sauvies Island, Oregon.

Elizabeth Eckstrom is Chief of Geriatrics in the Division of General Internal Medicine & Geriatrics at Oregon Health & Science University. Her research focuses on healthy aging and has shown that tai chi reduces falls by at least 50% and improves memory test scores (she recommends tai chi for everyone!). She is grateful to care for and learn from her older patients, and has had the opportunity to teach conferences and workshops on fall prevention and healthy aging around the world. She is thrilled to call Oregon home and can frequently be found in her garden, windsurfing on the Columbia River, and hiking and skiing on Mt. Hood.

"*The Gift of Aging* is itself a gift. It's packed with research-based strategies and motivating stories of elders that can help make growing older the most meaningful ride of a lifetime!"

Daniel H. Pink, author of *When, Drive,* and *To Sell Is Human*

"This is a beautiful book. *The Gift of Aging* is filled with lots of practical advice – but none more practical than "have a purpose.' The last decades of our lives can be the most important, productive, and fulfilling, but only if we take them with the seriousness (and the good humor) they deserve!'

Bill McKibben, author of *The End of Nature* and *The Flag, the Cross, and the Station Wagon*

"*The Gift of Aging* is a remarkable book that challenges us to look at aging not as a hopeless condition of wrinkled skin, immobility, and failing memory, but as an important and potentially healthy stage of life."

Daniel Gibbs, author of *A Tattoo on My Brain*

"I love how this inspiring and companionable book combines profound spiritual wisdom with utterly down-to-earth advice, marrying reflections on the deepest questions of life's meaning with recipes and financial planning tactics. Marcy Houle and Elizabeth Eckstrom show that while getting older is necessarily a process of becoming more aware of our human limitations, it's also an invitation to step more wholeheartedly *into* those limitations, becoming ever more fully the people we were meant to be. For the first time in a while, I find myself relishing the prospect of advancing age."

Oliver Burkeman, author of *Four Thousand Weeks: Time Management for Mortals*

By The Same Authors

The Gift of Caring: Saving Our Parents – and Ourselves – from the Perils of Modern Healthcare

Also By Marcy Houle

Wings for My Flight: The Peregrine Falcons of Chimney Rock
The Prairie Keepers: Keepers of the Zumwalt
A Generous Nature: Lives Transformed by Oregon
Forest Park: Exploring Portland's Natural Sanctuary

The Gift of Aging

Growing Older with Purpose, Planning, and Positivity

MARCY COTTRELL HOULE, MS
ELIZABETH ECKSTROM, MD, MPH, MACP

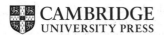

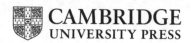

CAMBRIDGE
UNIVERSITY PRESS

Shaftesbury Road, Cambridge CB2 8EA, United Kingdom

One Liberty Plaza, 20th Floor, New York, NY 10006, USA

477 Williamstown Road, Port Melbourne, VIC 3207, Australia

314–321, 3rd Floor, Plot 3, Splendor Forum, Jasola District Centre, New Delhi – 110025, India

103 Penang Road, #05–06/07, Visioncrest Commercial, Singapore 238467

Cambridge University Press is part of Cambridge University Press & Assessment, a department of the University of Cambridge.

We share the University's mission to contribute to society through the pursuit of education, learning and research at the highest international levels of excellence.

www.cambridge.org
Information on this title: www.cambridge.org/9781009330770

DOI: 10.1017/9781009330725

First published 2023 (version 2, August 2023)

Printed in the United Kingdom by TJ Books Limited, Padstow Cornwall

A catalogue record for this publication is available from the British Library

A Cataloging-in-Publication data record for this book is available from the Library of Congress

ISBN   978-1-009-33077-0   Hardback
ISBN   978-1-009-33073-2   Paperback

. . . .

This book is lovingly dedicated to
Lilly Cohen
who remains the wind in the sails of Team Caring.

"What is the gift of aging? Seeking and finding beauty, where many people think beauty isn't. It is taking the time to stop, look, and listen.

"When you're young, you're so busy talking that you don't spend much time listening. But as you mature, you can learn to stand on top of all that talking, and become a listener. You have a context now for all that talk; what you hear is being added to a structure that's in place. You have developed inventory. And as you move through life that inventory piles up.

"When you hear talk, there is more reference for it now, more meaning and evaluation. And this is not merely talk in words. Rather, it is messages that are coming at you. Messages from people and from nature. You can look and see and listen to what the estuaries and trees are saying and the landscape of nature.

"The gift of aging is climbing higher and higher up this beautiful mountain that lets you see further and further each day in every way. The base gets wider and the pinnacle gets higher. And you get to stand on it at no charge, which is the beauty.

"Life experience has built the mountain you stand on. From here, you will find amazing discoveries because you can see far beneath you. The gift is not in answers, no. Instead, the gift is seeing a much bigger view of the questions, which is just as exciting.

"It becomes even more miraculous."

Neal Maine,
age 85

CONTENTS

TABLES

CONTRIBUTORS

Wendy K. Goidel, Esq., principal of Goidel Law Group PLLC, dedicates her practice to elder law and estate planning. Recognizing that elder law should not be practiced in a vacuum, Wendy developed and implemented Concierge Care Coordination®, an innovative, holistic practice model that seamlessly integrates geriatric social work with legal planning.

Wendy created fellowship programs at two New York universities designed to encourage social work students to enter the field of gerontology and promote collaboration between law and social work students. She gives back to the community and sponsors programs for individuals with cognitive impairment and their care partners. Wendy was honored for her contributions to several adult day programs in New York for individuals with cognitive impairment and was named as one of the Top 50 Women in Business by the Long Island Business News. For a decade, Wendy served on the Executive Board of Make-A-Wish, Suffolk County, NY.

Wendy is admitted to practice law in New York and Connecticut. She graduated from Cardozo School of Law where she served as Editor-in-Chief of the Cardozo Arts & Entertainment Law Journal. Wendy graduated magna cum laude from Syracuse University's S.I. Newhouse School of Public Communications.

Darla Phillips (PT, DPT, ATC, OCS, RRCA Certified Running Coach) graduated from the University of Southern California with a Doctorate of Physical Therapy (DPT). She holds a Bachelor of Science in Health and Human performance with a concentration in Athletic Training from George Fox University and has enjoyed working with a variety of teams, including gymnastics, track, basketball, and football. She remains a certified Athletic Trainer (ATC) and has a passion for long distance running. Following PT school, she completed the Southern California Kaiser Orthopedic Residency program and became a Board-Certified Specialist in Orthopaedic Physical Therapy (OCS) as recognized by the American Board of Physical Therapy Specialists. Darla continued her work in outpatient orthopedics in Los Angeles before returning to her home state of Oregon.

FOREWORD

What a pleasure to get to say a few words at the outset of this remarkable book. In its pages, you will meet people aging – not just gracefully but *gratefully*.

In a society – and world – as youth-focused as ours, it's easy for people as they get older to try and cling to how they've lived in the past. But it's important to realize that we have entirely new opportunities to embrace as we get older.

Above all, I think, we can figure out how to help shape our societies for those that come after us. We have several advantages in this regard. For one thing, in the United States, those of us in our older years now have a memory of a society that worked better. Take the environment, the issue that's absorbed most of my life. If you're in your 60s or 70s or 80s, you were around for the first Earth Day (maybe you marched in it – 10% of Americans did, the biggest demonstration in the country's history). And then you got to watch – within a year – as a bipartisan group of politicians enacted the Clean Air Act and the Clean Water Act, and created the Environmental Protection Agency. That kind of response seems unimaginable to young people now, who have known only a deeply polarized and dysfunctional society. But we know that, if we did it once, we can do it again.

And we have the tools, as older people, to make all the difference. There are so many of us – 70 million people over the age of 60 in the US alone (a population larger than that of France!), and 10,000 more added each day. Americans vote in huge numbers, which magnifies our potential political impact – politicians have to listen to us. Though not all of us are well off, our generations did end up with most of the country's financial resources, which means that Wall Street needs to listen as well.

We have time. And we have kids and grandkids, as do communities around the globe, who take that abstract notion of 'legacy' and make it very concrete. Your legacy is the world you leave behind for the people you love the most.

So as I read this wonderful book, full of advice about how to stay sound in mind and body, I think mostly of the things we should try to stay sound *for*. What a privilege it is to get to make a difference!

Perhaps a way of thinking about it is: no one really wants to be "elderly," with the frailty and incapacity that implies. But all of us should want to be *elders*, with the wisdom and engagement that the name conjures up. The people in this book testify that connection and relationship are keys to making these years the culmination of our lives. And when that connection and relationship can be in *service* – well, that's a life well lived!

Bill McKibben, founder Third Act

INTRODUCTION

Elizabeth Eckstrom, MD, MPH, MACP

When Marcy asked me to consider writing another book together, it took me by surprise. After writing *The Gift of Caring*, I was pretty certain I wouldn't write another book. It was a lot of work, and I thought I had shared just about everything I knew about growing older! But she had an experience that made her realize she needed to start thinking about aging *now*, not wait, as many of us do, believing it is still a long way off and we can confront it when it happens.

And then, I considered all the colleagues, patients, family members, and our amazing readers who have asked both of us questions – questions we didn't answer in our first book, but that are all pressing issues for older adults.

What about kidney disease in old age? I want to hear more about osteoporosis. What if I run out of money? Is assisted living the only option I have when I grow old – I'm not looking forward to assisted living! Should I be on more medication, or less? Most importantly, tell me how I can *prevent* disability and decline for as long as possible, and live a healthy, fulfilled, and joyous long life.

I realized we did need to write another book. So many of my patients ask "What is normal at 80, 90, 100?" I realized we need to describe the normal changes of aging and help our readers understand how they can successfully adapt to these changes. We need to explain how to reduce the risk of dementia, falls, fractures, frailty, and other problems common with aging. We need to illuminate how to best plan for our future. We need to frame aging to optimize health and well-being.

All of us face many challenges as we age. None of us has complete control of our aging process. But a positive attitude toward aging can actually increase our life expectancy by seven years. If we start now, we can harness the power of positivity and planning to ensure we feel the way Neal Maine does (Chapter 33) as he experiences the pinnacle of his life's mountain.

Healthy aging has been a hot topic recently. Baby boomers are turning 65 at startling rates. In the United States (US), 100 people hit this landmark every 13 minutes, and this trend is being replicated around the world. As authors experiencing aging in the US, this book is inevitably slanted toward the opportunities and challenges that exist there, but the stories and healthy aging concepts, suggestions, and strategies will hopefully resonate around the world, as we are indeed a global community who has to respect, honor, support, and love each other to ensure all of us can thrive together. This large and diverse baby boomer generation (to which Marcy and I both belong) is changing the face of aging around the world. We all wish to age gracefully and with continued purpose, loving relationships, and, as I see in my patients' expressions each day, avoid the worst fears we all share: Alzheimer Disease and related dementias, loss of mobility, and loss of independence. Trust me: remaining free of these conditions is not just luck. It requires careful attention from a young age. Recent research supports the idea that Alzheimer Dementia is actually a disease that begins in early childhood (when poor educational attainment, poor exercise and diet habits, and low socioeconomic status create vulnerability that increases the risk of dementia later in life).

Many books have already been written on the topic of healthy aging. Products from skin care to medical devices promise magical reversal of the effects of aging. And these promises are not all false! Many of us are still participating in sports, traveling, and working well into our 70s and later – acting 20 years younger than our parents did at the same age, and having the bodies and brains to go with it.

As a geriatrician and researcher who has specialized in the care of older adults for over 25 years, I believe aging well and with joy *is* a mantra everyone can adopt – whether we are rich or poor, have chronic illnesses or are completely healthy, and whether we have a large and supportive family or a much smaller social network.

Further, we need to do it as a community, not reserving aging well for the affluent or smartest people. The baby boom generation will only succeed into old age if we support aging well for our entire generation. Poverty, low education level, discrimination, and other social determinants of health make aging well challenging for many of us, our friends and neighbors. We need to work together to ensure that everyone has every opportunity to age well.

And so I told Marcy "yes." I would embark on this new expedition with her. This book is modeled after *The Gift of Caring* in that it shares some of Marcy's and my personal stories, stories of my patients and other older adults who are doing amazing things as they age, and then offers practical advice and strategies to assist each of us in enhancing our potential to age well.

It is interesting to note that most of the elders in this book were surprised when we approached them to tell their stories. They said, "there is nothing special about me!" They felt they were just living life; learning, engaging, and finding joy every day. Yet these are the stories that inspired Marcy and me, and we hope will inspire you as well.

To be fair: it isn't easy. We need to attend to physical, cognitive, psychological, and spiritual health every single day. We need to engage in purposeful activities – whether work, volunteering, or helping to care for others. We need to laugh, to be generous, to try new things at least once a week (how about French classes or Oaxacan food?), and make friends younger than we are (so they don't die before us). We need to have a positive attitude, discover new passions and follow them, and find ways we can give back and make a difference. And, most of all, we need to spend time with family, friends, and those who value our support to age just a little better.

The results are entirely worth it. It is possible, if we begin planning now, to thrive in our later years, and to live with joy until life's end. Marcy was shaken into awareness of what aging looks like. We hope this book will allow our readers to plan for their own futures without needing such a dramatic wake-up call!

1 MAP AND COMPASS

Marcy Cottrell Houle

Three months before starting this book I had a fall – a ridiculous fall, really, because I wasn't paying attention. That's the reason for many falls, I think. It happened in a Kroger parking lot when I was fiddling with the handles of my purse while hurrying toward the store entrance. I tripped on a drainage grate – and broke both my arms.

That's right, not just one, but what doctors call bilateral fractures, near the elbows. For a month I could not use either arm, which meant I could not do *anything*. I could not open a door, tie a shoelace, cut up my food, take a shower by myself, cut my nails, and, well, all the *other* things we take for granted we can do when we have hands and arms.

Thankfully, I have a spouse, John, who was able to take time off from work to care for me. Family members and friends were also there to help. I was lucky. In three months, I was back to normal. My arms had healed. I was independent again. I felt ready to move on with my life.

Wait. Not quite.

While I was grateful to think "nothing's changed," in truth, something had. For the first time, I saw what it felt like to be helpless, unable to care for myself. Even more humbling and distressing, at times I felt like a burden to the ones I loved the most.

What I had experienced is the ghost that looms ahead of all of us. Aging. My crisis, albeit a temporary one, was a wake-up call, a chance to stop the time wheel and peer into myself. And, in a strange, upside-down way, it was also a gift.

Broken bones a gift? Yes. Because with my incapacity came a reckoning I had purposely avoided, having constructed a virtual wall around myself.

Until I was 40, I never gave a thought to aging – that is, until my parents started getting sick. Then it came to the forefront of my life. But even so, it was about *them*, and their generation. Now, having suffered two broken arms and the inability to do all the things I took for granted, I realized the specter of aging is no longer about parents or old people.

It's about me.

Or will be before I know it. Even though everything healed well and doctors said I could resume all my normal activities, my accident cast a shadow. There would come a time when I would not be able to spring back and do all the things I loved to do.

I had seen my parents and their friends go through this stage. Soon, my group – those 60-somethings who are starting down this path with tens of thousands of others – will be standing in that same spotlight none of us wants to talk about, as we race to build higher walls around ourselves, frantically keeping the aging demons at bay.

The tearing down of that invisible barricade was a good thing for it gave me an unobstructed view. It allowed me to see – ever so faintly – the lay of the land stretching out ahead in new and curious ways. It made me want to know everything I could, in traveling this frontier, to be able to do it more purposefully, stronger, and better. I had seen my wonderful parents go through a fragmented and broken medical system that I didn't want to experience myself or have anyone I cared about endure.

Was it possible if one approached the journey in an intentional way to be excited about aging, about this chapter in life some very old people say is their happiest?

Their *happiest*? How could that be?

Elizabeth Eckstrom, my friend, co-author, and a geriatrician who has treated hundreds of older patients for 25 years, said many of her patients feel that way about the third and fourth chapters of their lives. They are *happy*. She herself is enthusiastic about aging. She is so excited about it, in fact, that she recently took nearly a year's sabbatical to travel around the world to research where people are aging the best.

The photos she brought home of older people intrigued me. They were a far cry from pictures of aged, wizened hands that my mother, who lived to be 93, always hated. Those stock images seemed to represent decline, frailty, a person inches from death, even when one might be years from the end. Whereas the photographs Elizabeth had with her were of 95-year-old Italians climbing ladders and pruning olive trees. All this after they had just walked 5 miles up and down cobblestone roads! Of course, she said that if we tried that in America, people would be falling from their ladders and breaking their hips. It took a lifetime of experience to learn how to stay steady on a ladder and prune trees.

Still, I liked those photographs. What they proffered was liveliness in old age. Now I wondered: Is liveliness really possible when we grow old? Here? In America? The answer seemed especially significant as, after my injury, I often felt fatigued. Moreover, most of us don't reside in a *Blue Zone* – those exceptional places that Elizabeth visited.

First studied by researcher Dan Buettner and his *National Geographic* team, Blue Zones are sites where a significant number of people live to be over 100 and are still in relatively good health. Buettner and his fellow researchers identified five Blue Zones in the world: Nuoro province in Sardinia, Italy; Nicoya, Costa Rica; Icaria, Greece; Okinawa, Japan; and the Seventh Day Adventist community of Loma Linda, California.

Centenarians in Blue Zone regions are not like other old people around the globe. They are largely free of the diseases that plague the rest of us; heart disease, depression, and diabetes are rare. Even more intriguing, Buettner found that the rate of dementia in these communities is extremely low. People in the Blue Zones develop dementia at a 75% lower rate than in the United States!

But what does this all mean for those of us who don't live in these extraordinary locations? Are there strategies that everyone – no matter what culture, population, region we live in – might engage in to enjoy some of the positive features of the Blue Zones closer to all our homes?

For nearly three decades, Elizabeth has sought to understand how people who are the happiest and healthiest live life through multiple lenses: medically, physically, emotionally, psychologically, spiritually. Part of her drive is that she knows the answers for America can't come quickly enough. Because the statistics in the literature are grim. And they aren't, she explains, just about old people.

In the 2022 Bloomberg *Healthiest Country Index*, the United States ranked a depressing #34 in its Health Grade (and it continues to go down every year), scoring below Estonia, Chile, Cuba, and *just above* Bahrain and Qatar. In a recent article in the *Journal of General Internal Medicine*, researchers conclude that (a) the United States has the most expensive, technologically advanced, and sub-specialized healthcare system in the world, and yet (b) a *worse population health status than any other high-income country*.

This situation poses special problems for older adults, says Elizabeth. Added to that are "happiness indexes." The United States places low on those too. Other countries have much higher "happiness indexes" and older persons are healthier and more contented as they age.

According to the World Happiness Report, the annual survey by the Sustainable Development Solutions Network for the United Nations, of the 20 happiest countries in 2022, the US ranked number 16.

Why? I ask. Is there anything we can do about that?

Elizabeth thinks there is. But it starts long before one gets old. Our health and well-being at 80 are dependent on how we have lived our lives in the decades before. Yet, she adds, even at 80 there are still things we can do to make later years productive and joyous.

Happiness for individuals is dictated by several things, says Elizabeth: 40% of happiness is dictated by our genes; 15% by life circumstances; 40% is *under our own control*. Scientists aren't sure what accounts for the remainder of happiness.

But 40% is a powerful number.

Daniel Pink, the author of *Drive*, studies intrinsic motivation. The research he cites, while primarily directed toward business, also pertains to powerful ways to grow older. Grit, says Pink, is essential. Effort, too, is needed. Successful living is a three-legged stool. It requires a sense of purpose, of mastery, and of autonomy.

Interestingly, Elizabeth elucidates that all three are pivotal to keeping our brains healthy as we age. Understanding them, planning for them, can bring joy in our older years – and, indeed, right up until the time we die.

With the aging wall now broken down after my accident, these insights suddenly seemed more important than ever. The journey is one I want to learn about and I'm eager to embark. All that's missing is a map. That I would have to make. And I would need compass headings. Elizabeth could supply those. I knew there would be fallen trees to climb over, roots on the path to trip over, difficult stream crossings. That was okay with me if I had an idea what lay ahead and a notion of what the mountain top looked like.

Elizabeth would be an excellent guide. She has led hundreds up this path, and is up to date on trail conditions, having long examined, explored, and discovered some of the best treks up the mountain, while always on the lookout for a safer, more beautiful route. While she faces forward much of the time, Elizabeth also turns around to inspect and mark where the pitfalls have been hidden along the way.

Why? Because that, as Elizabeth explains, is what aging truly is. It's not, as we normally think, a range of dates or something that happens as you get old. And it's not one straight line. Aging is a continuum, a process.

For me, thinking of it that way makes the whole trajectory seem less sinister. Aging is the same path I've been on since I was small. It doesn't mean young. It doesn't mean old. What's more, it doesn't mean those pictures of shriveled hands. It is a comprehensive, undulating, moving line, with dates and years merely acting as markers on the route. Much of it is friendly. The path has been my partner for a long time.

The difference, as Elizabeth says, is that some things *do* change along that line. Challenges arise. But we get to choose how we are going to face them. There are positive ways to care for our mind, our body, and our soul. And to cultivate the vitality of each.

I just had to figure them out and put them on my map.

Two broken arms did that. They brought to light a stark realization and changed the meaning of aging for me. The wisdom of elders to teach me how to live meaningfully and well, twined with the knowledge of experts, is no longer a vague and indeterminate quest or a journey to a land of passivity and devolution.

It is the most alive thing I can imagine.

"Come to my office next Tuesday," Elizabeth says. "There's someone I'd like you to meet."

PART I
Caring For Your Mind

You want to know the secret to finding joy? Every day, I try to make life a little better for someone else. Then, the joy comes.

Rabbi Josh Stampfer,
age 97

2 A GOAL HIGHER THAN JOY

Marcy Cottrell Houle

The man happily chatting with Elizabeth in her office looks up from his wheelchair when I enter. Immediately I notice his smile stretches ear to ear. He reaches out his hand to shake mine. Knowing his advanced age, I extend my hand, expecting a fragile grip.

My fingers are crushed.

"Marcy," says Elizabeth, grinning, "I'd like you to meet Rabbi Josh Stampfer."

"Please, call me Josh," he says, his kind brown eyes putting me instantly at ease.

From an earlier conversation with Elizabeth, I know that Josh, at nearly 98, has lived a remarkable life. Welcomed to join the group, I take the vacant chair next to him. On Josh's other side is his caregiver, who outstretches her arm to shake my other hand. There is palpable warmth in this confab, I sense, and I think back to what Elizabeth had told me about this generous and well-loved man.

Born in Jerusalem in 1921 to a pioneering family in Israel, Josh's early years were surrounded by rabbis. His great-grandfather had been the chief rabbi of Jerusalem, founding one of the first Jewish settlements in Palestine when it was ruled by the Ottoman Empire. Josh's father, too, became a rabbi, also serving in Ottoman-controlled Palestine.

After World War I, with the fall of the Ottoman Empire, the government in Palestine was left in limbo. In 1922, the League of Nations approved British control of Palestine. For Josh's father, it was a time of scarce work. When Josh was 2 years old, the family left for America, where his father became a rabbi in a number of cities across the country.

Josh followed in his family's footsteps. Attending the Jewish Theological Seminary in New York City, in 1949 he was ordained as a rabbi. Four years later, desiring to see the West Coast, he took a position in Portland, Oregon. It would become his lifelong home, and from this base Josh would impact hundreds of lives in Portland, the entire Pacific Northwest – even the world.

Three years after arriving in Oregon, the rabbi established a retreat and education center – Camp Solomon Schechter – serving and prized by thousands of children, Jewish as well as those of other religions. Over 60 years later, it is still thriving. As a spiritual leader, Josh spent years traveling the world, in China, Birobidzhan, and Russia, to establish contact with Jewish people living in remote locations and facing dire conditions. Closer to home, Josh was a congregational rabbi from 1954 to 1993. He established the Oregon Holocaust Resource Center, built the Oregon Jewish Historical Society, and helped found the Oregon Jewish Museum. He'd also been a professor at Portland State University for 40 years, and established the Institute for Judaic Studies.

I am captivated by his story. Even more, I'm awed that, considering his age and obvious health issues, he doesn't appear to be satisfied, closing in on 100, to live a life of quiet retirement.

"All older persons have a capacity to continue to live a vibrant life, with joy and purpose," he says, smiling, when Elizabeth asks him about it. "You just have to make sure that you're not merely going to *enjoy* life. There is a goal higher than joy."

Higher than joy? A bit startled, I think of all the people I know eager to retire from work and start a sprint to enjoy life. Many wish to race to travel to as many places as possible, eat at the trendiest restaurants, look terrific, always seeking that next great adventure. Why? Because we are told all those things bring happiness. And we better get doing them before it's too late for us. Yet this is not what Josh was saying or the way he had chosen to spend his golden years.

The rabbi resettles himself in his wheelchair, reclines slightly, then explains.

"The goal in my life is to try to improve the lives of others. It is hoping to instill morality, ethics, and goodness into life. It is hoping to make our world a little better for everyone."

"How do you pursue that now?" Elizabeth asks.

"Through teaching. If I didn't teach, I wouldn't be sitting here. More importantly, I would be miserable."

The rabbi details his vigorous teaching schedule. "This morning I had a class of 55 students. I teach a history class one day a week. I also teach the Talmud once a week. One day a month, which will be tomorrow, I teach Jewish concepts to a group of men. For this class we will be discussing the issues of immigration, which are enormous. You know what the solution is?" he asks, with a glance at me. I shake my head, amazed at his vigor. "To improve the life of people elsewhere so that they want to continue to live there. The majority of people naturally want to live at home. They love their home. We have to help.

"When I founded the Institute for Judaic Studies at Portland State University 40 years ago, it was the only center for Middle East studies for undergraduate education in the country. It wasn't just Jewish, taught by Jewish professors," he explains. "We had Muslim and Christian teachers, too. It was all very interreligious; it was everyone working together. Which is what we should be doing now. We need to learn to live together. We need to respect each other's traditions. We need to see ourselves as part of a greater whole."

He pauses for a brief moment. "We take care of ourselves by taking care of others. We must learn we are not solitary beings. We are part of the wonderful community of humanity."

"Teaching and learning are great avocations when we grow older," I conclude.

"They are two different things," he clarifies. "Learning is an *avocation*. I love to learn! More and more people are learning in their adult years, and it's fun! Teaching, though, is a *vocation*. I have always taught. I have to keep it up. So I end up reading things that normally I would not be reading, knowing I have to prepare for a lecture. This is stimulating, because I know if I'm not prepared, I'm going to be embarrassed. The difference is, if I don't go to a movie, that means I don't go to a movie. If I don't read a book, that means I don't read a book. But if I am responsible for something, I am going to do it. As you grow older, I believe it is very important to be responsible *to* something or *for* something."

I have been searching for a definition of purpose and Josh has just nailed it.

"In all of us, there is an innate need for happiness," he reflects from over nine decades of experience. "But happiness is not just based on good health; not everyone has that. There is more to it. What I have found, and suggest to others: the way to be happy is to be good. Being good will make you happier. When people do a good deed for others, they really enjoy life more. It's very nice to have wonderful thoughts. But it's also important to translate those thoughts either into deeds or into words. Bringing happiness to others is the quickest way to have it yourself."

The old rabbi smiles again. His beaming countenance could brighten any dark room.

"So you are happy," Elizabeth says, smiling back.

"You know? I have become happier later in life, and I will tell you why. I love people. I just love people. I enjoy getting to know people and exploring ideas with people. That is why I love teaching; it brings me into contact with people. I encourage everyone, as they grow older, to use your skills."

"What if you don't think you have any, say, when you're 70, 80, 90?" I interject, thinking of a depressing article I recently read citing you will have made all your life contributions by age 75. The author wanted to die before reaching 80.

"Think you don't have any skills when you're older or anything to offer? Of course you do!" Josh exclaims. "Everybody develops skills during their lifetime. The point is to *transmit* them. You may have to look for opportunities; sometimes you have to *create* the opportunities after you retire. But you can always draw upon your own experience to help others."

He takes the thought a bit deeper. "It is true, there is always the desire to feel sorry for yourself. It's easy to turn in on yourself. Don't do it. A self-centered attitude is a major source of unhappiness. When you focus too much on yourself, you become disconnected from others. When you dwell only on your own needs and wants, it leads to insecurity and anxiety. You have to learn to overcome that."

"How do you do that?" I ask, thinking how easy it was to slip into feeling sorry for myself when grappling with two broken arms.

"Really, the answer is simple," Josh replies. "Take yourself out of yourself. How much better it is to do good for others. Think more in terms of what you can do to improve another person's life, and then, *go do it!*"

The old rabbi's grin is filled with warmth and I am moved to listen closely to his words. Here is a man, nearing a century in age, who has faced serious illness, the loss of his beloved life partner of nearly 70 years, seen Jewish communities in different parts of the world surviving under the most difficult circumstances, yet can honestly say he still loves life.

"You want to know the secret to finding joy?" says Josh, with a serenity I envied. "Every day, I try to make life a little better for someone else. Then, the joy comes."

3 WHY DOES HAVING PURPOSE MATTER?

Elizabeth Eckstrom, MD, MPH, MACP

While visiting the Nuoro Province in Sardinia off the coast of Italy, I noticed something fascinating. In the picturesque city streets, bustling squares, and remote mountains, a remarkable phenomenon caught my attention ... striking in that it was not something I would expect to see at home.

On a seemingly average weekday morning, I observed well-dressed men, often in suit and tie, moving quickly and casually. On their way to work, they interacted with everyone they passed on the cobblestone streets. They appeared relaxed and smiled during their conversations.

The thing was: these men were 80, 90, even 100 years old.

They live in one of the world's "Blue Zones" – places in the world with the highest number of centenarians, or people who have lived to be over 100. Dan Buettner and his team of researchers from *National Geographic* found nine factors that explained the amazing health and longevity of these regions. One became very clear to me while I visited and was something Josh Stampfer told Marcy. The centenarians of Nuoro Province know exactly what the rabbi is talking about: there *is* a goal higher than joy.

Purpose.

The older people of Sardinia, both men and women, care for themselves so they can also care for those they love. Women wear stylish dresses and high heeled shoes (something I do not recommend!) even on cobblestone streets. Men often are in groups, standing around chatting or arguing. They are the ones doing nearly all the shopping at the market, often shopping together, and are especially particular about selecting their vegetables, to the point of requesting the purveyors clean them and peel off damaged layers so they only pay for the best parts! They purchase sizable quantities of vegetables as if planning to cook a meal for a large family gathering.

Even more astonishing when I consider how many Americans rush to shop at convenience stores, shopping for vegetables in Sardinia can take most of the morning.

In spring when I visited, I observed these older men walking, cane-free, along cobblestone roads, sometimes travelling miles to their place of work: olive plantations, where their job is to prune olive trees. After trekking, they climb into the trees or onto step ladders, holding hand clippers or small saws, to trim the branches. Sometimes there are up to four people to a tree, sometimes still in suit jackets! They were completely engaged in meaningful work to support their families.

These Blue Zone Italians are doing far more risky physical activity than people in their 80s and 90s do in the United States. While I do not advise my older patients to climb ladders (absolutely not! – unless you have been doing it consistently for the last 80 years, of course), I do encourage them to live like the Sardinians, engaging in purposeful socializing and purposeful work.

Daniel Pink, author of *Drive*, could not agree more with this. He writes: "Humans, by their nature, seek purpose, to make a contribution and to be a part of a cause greater and more enduring than themselves." For older people in Nuoro Province, that greater cause is the well-being of their family, their community, and their environment. They are walking, working, interacting – with purpose.

This intrinsic motivation is also evident in the Okinawan Blue Zone. Older people here also demonstrate a strong sense of purpose. It is called *ichigai*, or "essentials for happiness." It is the reason people get up every morning. It may be to care for grandchildren, work in their garden, cook for their family, or other undertakings, but these simple tasks are profound – they foster a strong sense of purpose.

Unfortunately, many of us in America and elsewhere in the world do not have these anchoring responsibilities to help us maintain purpose in our lives. But there are things we can do to create this essential element and vastly improve our chance for health, fitness, and joy as we age. Understanding the critical role that having a purpose brings to our lives is the place to start.

Purpose can take many shapes, from raising a garden full of fresh produce, to helping to care for grandchildren, to volunteering at the local historical society, to starting a whole new encore career! The key to finding purpose is to be doing something – not just for yourself – but for others.

Actions You Can Take
1   Always ask WHY you are doing what you are doing.
2   If what you are doing has no purpose, or a purpose you are not passionate about, think about how you can change your behavior to make it more purposeful.
3   Reflect on what you are interested in. Maybe you have always wanted to mentor underserved teens. Maybe you would like to learn more about sustainable gardening.
4   Look around you to see who needs your support.
5   Reach out to your community – whether it be the library or your local parks and recreation office – to find out where you can contribute your skills, energy, and inspiration.
6   And, most importantly, don't wait. *Dive in!* You will be appreciated and, as Rabbi Josh Stampfer tells us, then the joy comes, when you try to make life a little better for someone else.

Besides bringing satisfaction, I tell my patients that when we have a purpose, it gives us something for which to get up in the morning!

AN OPEN AND
DETERMINED
MINDSET

Each day we have is a gift.... Life is full of highs and lows. Gratitude for the good things in our life is very important.... It counterbalances the inevitable problems, difficulties, and sorrows we all experience at times. If we can learn to adapt as we grow old, it allows us to find a new fullness of joy.

Lilly Cohen,
age 94

4 AN OPEN AND DETERMINED MINDSET

Marcy Cottrell Houle

"I would not be here now if not for a crying baby. She was the miracle we needed."

Lilly Cohen, a pretty, sprightly, well-dressed woman who, at 90, looks 10 years younger than her age, calmly sits before me drinking a cup of coffee. The challenges she has faced in life are inevident in her countenance and manner. Her thoughtful conversation helps me understand some of the reasons she has aged so well, which strike me as being especially valuable considering the hurdles life brought to her.

"As we travel through years, most of us know that changes in our lives are inevitable. Some of us take on the challenge of either preparing for them or dealing with them as they come along. Those who are successful are willing to make the necessary alterations to their current lifestyle to make the future easier to manage," she says. "We all desire to direct our own lives, even when you're 90. But to do that, it's all about," Lilly pauses momentarily, making sure I comprehend her emphasis, "*adaptability*."

I have learned a bit about adaptability – or lack of it – when I could not use my arms for a month. Rather than feel self-governing, I was captive to immobile casts, and required help with everything that previously I could easily do, including feeding myself. Very quickly I saw the value of autonomy – or the capacity to be independent. Lilly was right; it is something humans crave, though we may not recognize it until we are deprived of it.

"I first experienced change when I was 9 years old," she continues, "although it wouldn't be until years later when other trials arose that I would see the importance of being open to revising what you think is your life's course. Anticipating and planning adjustments to your everyday way of doing things can make a tremendous difference in your well-being. Of course, there are times in life when you have little choice, but the ability to adapt to changing circumstances is what will allow for triumph in life and," she adds, wisely, "success in aging. Your mindset will ultimately determine whether you view your life as one of despair or of gratitude."

Lilly's life certainly underscores how circumstances can bring changes that one could never expect.

Lilly shares that she was born in 1929 in a lovely part of Germany – Elberfeld-Wuppertal – a flourishing valley town in the Rhineland. Secure in a loving family, her father made a comfortable living in the men's clothing business he had founded with a partner, after leaving his homeland of Poland. He was well respected in the community. Smart and curious, she greatly enjoyed learning at her elementary school, where she was the only Jewish child in attendance.

"I experienced no antisemitism whatsoever," she declares.

Then came October 26, 1938, when her life changed forever.

"On that day, Adolf Hitler had decided on an '*Aktion*,' or action to expel the 18,000 Polish Jews living in Germany," she says, levelly. "The Polish consul in Düsseldorf, a city close by, who knew my parents, called to warn my father that something terrible was about to happen. Thinking that the danger was only to Jewish men, he offered to hide my father in the Polish Consulate, while my mother, younger sister, and I could remain at home. My sister at the time was 10 months old."

Lilly's family reacted quickly. Her father left for Düsseldorf to remain safe. But the consul was mistaken. Hitler's action pertained to *all* Polish Jews.

"Not long after my father left, two storm troopers came to our door," Lilly continues. "They said they were there to pick up all three of us, including the baby, who was the only Jewish infant in Elberfeld at that time. While we were being swiftly escorted from our home, not knowing where they were taking us, our housekeeper, a Christian from Czechoslovakia, whispered to my mother, 'Don't take any bottles of milk or diapers.' My mother followed her advice. We were taken to a local prison."

What happened next Lilly remembers vividly.

"There were over 200 Jewish people all crammed together, everyone nervous, not knowing what to expect. My baby sister, now famished and wet, began to cry. Then she started to scream. Then wail, non-stop. The fastidious Nazi manager of this Jew-gathering operation became increasingly annoyed. He ordered her to quit crying. But nothing can stop a hungry, screeching baby. Finally, unwilling to stand a moment more of the squealing, he ordered the storm troopers who had brought us to prison to take us back home. He was also furious that my father was missing.

Lilly pauses before continuing, remembering a very painful part of her life. "The next morning, all the Polish Jews that we had seen in the prison were loaded into box cars, taken to the Polish border and expelled from Germany," she says. "Once in Poland, they were housed in temporary camps in Lodz, a central city in the country. As we were to learn later, most of the Jews driven out from Germany during the Aktion later died in the Lodz Ghetto or were sent on to concentration camps where they were exterminated.

"My family was lucky. We were able to escape and meet up with my father in Paris. He had obtained visas to Cuba and the United States. We left Europe at the end of December in 1938, and sailed to Havana, where we lived as refugees for a year and a half. We came to New York in July 1940. Unfortunately, my mother's family lost 25 people to the Holocaust in Poland. Our fast-thinking housekeeper, and my sister's unstoppable wailing, had been our miracles."

Listening to Lilly renders me speechless. With a blend of peace and poise, she finishes her story.

"Twenty-six other members of our family, however, survived. Today, they live all over – in France, Holland, Israel, Canada, and the United States. Thankfully, all our family have grown and flourished in the years that followed."

The lessons of adaptation Lilly acquired as a child stayed with her as she continued her life in New York. She attended college. Years later, she received a Master's degree in Higher and Adult Education and also studied Gerontological Practice. She married a wonderful man, had two children, and soon found her academic experience called to the front lines, when her ailing mother-in-law came to live with their family. Not long after, her beloved husband declined from a neurological disease, undiagnosed for 10 years.

"George developed cognitive, physical, and emotional losses which caused premature aging. I was to become his caregiver for 20 years," Lilly relates. "My ability to cope and to survive was helped immeasurably by my local Well Spouse support group, and later by my activism and then presidency of the national Well Spouse Association. Now that I am an old person myself, learning to live through loss and adapting to change are two concepts that continue to influence my thinking."

She is quick to add, however, that her life has not been just one of loss. Years after her husband died, she met her second husband, who, like her, was a spousal caregiver for many years. Together, they have formed a new life and found a deep and abiding love. With optimism, Lilly states her health is good, and they enjoy living in a Naturally Occurring Retirement Community (NORC) where there is an endless round of interesting activities that one can engage in. Today, she is intimately involved with Hofstra University's PEIR Program, or Personal Enrichment in Retirement – a lifelong learning program whose members range in age from their mid-50s to their late 90s. It is a community of older adults who value intellectual and cultural stimulation in a friendly social environment on a college campus.

"Interacting with several hundred retirees has given me the opportunity to study aging from many standpoints," Lilly – always an educator – reflects. "I began learning about aging and longevity in 1975 when I was 46, when my employer, the President of Adelphi University, asked me to establish a Multidisciplinary Center on Aging. Now I see it from my own perspective, as a person in her 90s and through multiple lenses. Probably the most valuable thing I've found is the importance of planning ahead. Denial of the aging process – unwillingness to consider the possibility of personal decline or loss – and refusal to think about the future and the contingencies related to aging, keep you from making any helpful arrangements."

Lilly reaches for her purse and pulls out her iPhone and glasses. "Speaking for myself and Al, we forget often where we put these things! We are less energetic, less steady on our feet, less adept at multi-tasking. All of this requires a shift in our thinking, *more* planning ahead.

"I see two types of people when they get to my age," she concludes.

I can't help smiling. "What are those, Lilly?"

"The *Denialists* and the *Realists*. Sometimes we can be a mixture of both. Denialists tend to be the more fearful and rigid folks whom I encounter, who insist on maintaining the status quo. Their denial gives them a sense of control. They believe they can and must continue to do what they have always done and maintain their usual lifestyle. They cannot accept the possibility of physical or mental weakness, health decline, or other losses. They dread thinking about these possibilities. What this means, when serious problems arise, is they are unprepared."

Lilly takes a sip of coffee. Her words make me realize how completely *unprepared* I was for the recent accident that changed my life momentarily, but altered my thinking even more. Of course, we can't prepare for an accident we don't know we are going to encounter; that's why those of us who can, have health insurance. But what Lilly is saying was that it *is* possible to prepare for life changes that will indeed come to all of us.

"Realists are able to view life as it actually is," she says, continuing her thought. "They anticipate some of the constructive changes they need to make for a positive old age. They are willing to make the necessary alterations to their current lifestyle to make the future easier to manage. That is how they maintain control – by *making adjustments now, sooner than later*, in advance of when they may be needed. Realists take action with an open and determined mindset to face life with foresight and courage when they can still handle the change."

"You are a realist, Lilly," I say, with admiration.

"Well, there are certainly some things I am very glad I've done, and they can be undertaken by all older people. No matter how old you are, you can still change what you think and what you do."

Lilly puts away her iPhone, and breaks into a smile.

"We all slow down as we grow old, but that isn't all bad. When your activities become more limited because of infirmity, you can focus on the things you can *still* do that give you the most pleasure! Think about them. Is it socializing with your family? Attending religious services? Cooking in or eating out? Playing cards or taking part in a university lifelong learning program, doing volunteer work, reading or watching television? Whatever it is, make sure you engage in activities that make you happy!

"In a long life we all have experienced pain, suffering, loss, and disappointment," she adds, thoughtfully. "But we have also had fun, joy, success, and memorable experiences. If we look at our past, and then regard our situation today, we can usually find things to be proud and happy about. Too many older people forget to do that! They get caught up in what they perceive to be their current misery. They focus only on loss and frustration. That's unfortunate."

Looking directly at my face, Lilly then says something I want on my map: "As we grow old, it's important to maintain a perspective on the *totality of life*. We need to try to remember the good luck we've had in the past, and the positives that remain in our current life. Because if we look deep inside ourselves, we *all* have positives in our lives. The important thing? Count your blessings!"

One good fortune of monumental significance came to Lilly last year. She was aware that the German government and local groups had begun acknowledging their country's terrible history and had gone public about it. Many German towns were inviting back the Jews who had fled. Those who had lived in Elberfeld-Wuppertal were invited to return for a three-day visit in April 2018. Mayors of cities were reaching out also to descendants of Jews who had to flee.

While some in her family were too frail to attend, and others could not afford the trip, and still others simply could not bear the thought of ever setting foot on German soil again, Lilly, at 88 years old, went, along with her daughter Susan, her grand-daughter Wendy, her cousin and his wife, and her husband Al.

Jews came to Elberfeld-Wuppertal from all parts of the world. They were invited to receptions, with speeches and presentations, all in German "which unfortunately I did not fully understand," she says with a slight tilt to her head. She was taken to the site of her former home, now a parking garage.

As she describes it, I find it amazing Lilly does not evince any sadness upon seeing the change to the lovely apartment building of her childhood. Instead, she shows me a picture of herself smiling with Al with obvious delight to be back at her initial home. The photo was printed in the local newspaper.

"What I learned from this trip was a better understanding of my parent's lives and my own life. It was an emotional experience," she says. "I'm thankful that the Jews of Elberfeld-Wuppertal and their stories have not been lost or forgotten. Most of all, it reinforced my belief that my family and I were so fortunate.

"Each day we have is a gift. And the gift of aging is perspective and experience. Life is full of highs and lows. Gratitude for the good things in our life is very important. Gratitude impacts our thoughts and feelings. It counterbalances the inevitable problems, difficulties, and sorrows we all experience at times. If we can learn to adapt as we grow old, it allows us to find a new fullness of joy."

Lilly, I know, has faced many bullets head-on in her life, including one she did not speak about today, and perhaps her greatest loss – the death of her beloved son from leukemia at age 49. Yet, somehow, she has withstood them all, and today sits erect across from me with a genuine belief that life is still good. No, not just good, but *very* good.

"Ultimately, happiness comes from the inside, not the outside," says Lilly. "It is understanding that each of us is a precious human life.

"I am so grateful my sister cried. Every single day, I pause to count my blessings."

5 AUTONOMY
Impossible without Adaptability

Elizabeth Eckstrom, MD, MPH, MACP

Centenarians tend to be decisive. They know what they want and then stay on course. But when life circumstances force them to adapt, they become flexible thinkers, able to embrace the change. And, they are likeable.

This quote from the Blue Zone of Okinawa, Japan, really says it all. People who live long and well have set a course for themselves. If life throws them a punch, though, they figure out how to roll with it.

How can we learn from these wise elders to maintain our autonomy through adaptability? Let's look at what they can teach us.

First of all, they recognize *change is inevitable*. We all know that truth in our hearts, though some of us would prefer to believe otherwise. That is what makes aging so hard for so many. We see ourselves changing as we age, but we prefer to *ignore* the changes rather than learn as much as we can about them. By pretending them away, we lose the opportunity to adapt proactively and become successful in those changes.

Making positive choices is what this book is about – if you are reading it, you are already on a good path to aging well! Understanding the changes we must adapt to as we age helps us maintain greater control of them – such as voluntarily giving up driving before having an accident and learning the public transportation system if you have macular degeneration.

In essence, it boils down to: we can either *act to maintain control* as much as possible during change, or we can let changes *occur to us* – which often leads to pain, loss of function, and loss of independence.

Studies show maintaining autonomy is linked to well-being. Making constructive adjustments to preserve our autonomy will help us age well.

Here is an illustration. For someone who has little family support and worsening Parkinson Disease, maintaining autonomy does *not* mean remaining in your own home and possibly suffering a fall and hip fracture. Rather, it could mean reviewing financial means and then choosing an alternative – whether it be in employing home care assistance or moving to an assisted living or continuing care environment.

By recognizing the need to make a change, you can control the team you employ, the residence to which you move, and the way you settle in to this new environment. Waiting for the fall and hip fracture might mean a hurried move to a facility that you have not chosen yourself, but in which you will spend the rest of your life.

Maintaining autonomy often means *accepting some risk*. One of my favorite quotes from the noted surgeon and author Atul Gawande is "We want autonomy for ourselves and safety for those we love." People whose goal is to remain independent for as long as possible may put themselves in problematic situations.

We need to assess each situation, determine the current risk, and act to maintain as much autonomy as possible within the context of whatever health challenge is threatening autonomy.

For example, patients with advanced dementia often develop problems eating and swallowing. I help families and caregivers learn to assist them to eat as safely as possible, knowing the patient may have aspiration of food into their lungs. There is risk in that, of course, but it allows them to retain the joy and ritual of eating. Good research shows that feeding tubes do not improve quantity or quality of life in persons with dementia, so assisted feeding is the much better option.

I often suggest these ten action strategies to my patients to enhance well-being as we age:

• Be realistic. You will slow down. That's okay. Understand the need to make less ambitious social and activity plans.

- Recognize this slower pace is not something to be avoided or dreaded. It can bring with it new and deeper meaning to the things you enjoy.
- Collect information about resources and services that are designed for older adults, such as transportation assistance, emergency health services, and recreation options. These will be valuable as you adjust to your changing body.
- Join support groups and lifelong learning programs, do volunteer work, engage in social events. These improve one's quality of life.
- Take advantage of the digital world to communicate with grandchildren and friends, shop from home, and utilize well-being and other great apps.
- Learn how to use new gadgets (e.g., low vision aids or a "smart" medication reminder) which make it possible to navigate the world in different ways (but be careful not to succumb to gimmicks).
- When digital devices and gadgets seem overwhelming, ask for help from your grandchildren or other young persons to assist you in figuring them out! This comes easy to them and they can enjoy being helpful to you.
- Don't wait for "red flags" like crashes, scrapes on the car, new medical diagnoses, or worsening health conditions to stop driving. Start early in identifying other transportation options.
- *Realize early* when you need more help. Reach out for help when something requires lifting, bending, or climbing ladders.
- Make your home or apartment safe to reduce the chance of falling.

Adapting to changes that come with aging can be viewed as an opportunity to discover new things about yourself. As Lilly Cohen shows us, keeping an open and determined mindset, and facing life with foresight and courage, can allow us to embrace each stage and make it the best it can possibly be.

One thing … important to a good long life is a sense of humor. It helps take us through all sorts of life's turns and twists, if we can nurture that. Laughter is good for the soul. We need to have fun together, first; then occasionally along life's path, the only solution is just to be able to laugh at yourself.

Lucille Pierce,
age 101

6 DANCE, LUCILLE, DANCE

Marcy Cottrell Houle

"Mastery is a pain," says researcher Daniel Pink.

Yet it is also a prime motivator that helps us stretch ourselves to become better at something we care about. And having passion for goals, whatever they are, gives meaning to our lives. The problem is, mastery takes time and patience, and – here's the word again that keeps coming up – grit.

Grit means we must personally show effort. It doesn't come automatically, like streaming movies. It entails working and working at something, even when we don't see much advancement, which is most of the time. Yet what it offers is a sense of engagement, a validation that we are trying to do something that matters to us and hoping, over time, to improve.

Attempting mastery in anything can feel frustrating. That's *okay*. It's part of developing a growth mindset – the ability to learn from your mistakes and treat them as opportunities for growth. Infuse that growth mindset with emotional intelligence and you have a winning formula for mastery. Having something to care about and wanting to get better at is a crucial part of aging well and healthfully. Even more compelling, as Elizabeth says, this is all very, very good for our brains.

But I didn't learn about this from a book.

I learn about mastery from Lucille.

Meeting at her home to have lunch, I notice all around Lucille Pierce's apartment are examples of beautiful calligraphy – hanging on the walls, framed on tables, with unfinished art pieces lying on desks.

"Art is a joyous thing," says Lucille, smiling, welcoming me inside. "It is very satisfying to be able to create something tangible.

So many things are not definite and physical, and so much now is electronic. When computers first came into our lives, I was determined not to use them!" She laughs. "Now, of course, I see their worth. But I am a creative person; I want to make things myself! What is so wonderful about art is you can shape something that can give others joy.

"It's really more of a hobby," she says, as if to clarify. "It's something I just love to do. And I'm fortunate that I still have a steady hand."

This is no hobby, I posit, following Lucille toward her cozy dining area, and I am anxious to learn more.

Lucille entered my life through a fortuitous ripple effect. A friend of hers – a calligraphy artist – wrote to tell me how much Lucille had enjoyed *The Gift of Caring*. She had given the book to her. Her friend also wrote that Lucille, in turn, gave *The Gift of Caring* to her daughters.

"Lucille feels so good because her daughters told her that, after having read your book, they will never let what your parents went through happen to her. They have been forewarned, and are prepared to be her advocates! Lucille is 98 years old, and an artist, though she won't call herself that. She is a beautiful calligrapher, still takes classes, and lives on her own. She is a wonderful role model for me."

I decided I wanted to meet Lucille for myself. What does a 98-year-old calligrapher look like? What did it mean that she still takes classes? What is life like for a near-centenarian artist?

Her friend set up the meeting. Lucille said she wanted to meet me at her apartment and would treat me to lunch. When I remonstrated that I didn't want her to go to extra effort, her friend said, "That is just the way she is. Giving. You'll see. Ask her about her knitting projects for homeless people."

Knitting for the homeless? Now I had no idea what to expect.

"I hope you like tuna," Lucille says, as we move across the sunny room, past her studio. Lucille catches my eye peeking in the room where there is a large, paper banner taped high on the wall. It reads, "Dance, Lucille, Dance."

Lucille laughs. "*I* didn't create that. One of my granddaughters made it as a surprise for my 90th birthday and her husband hung it there without me knowing. Obviously, I could not take it down! It makes me happy seeing it and thinking about that great party!"

She leads me to the dining table, which Lucille has prettily set. There is fresh fruit, bread, jam and butter, and two plates of Salade Nicoise, with albacore tuna, red-skinned potatoes, and thin green beans. A pitcher of cold water with ice sits on the table, ready to be poured into glasses. A vase of cheerful yellow daffodils rests as a happy centerpiece decoration.

"Lucille, I feel as if I've been invited to tea at the Empress Hotel in Victoria!" I reply, astonished at the work she has expended to make all this come together.

"It's the least I can do for you, now that you have prepared my family, after reading *The Gift of Caring*, to save me from 'the perils of modern healthcare.'" She smiles, and passes me what looks to be homemade jam. "I enjoy making my own meals. I think I got that from my parents, who both grew up on farms. My father had a wonderful garden. That's what kept people eating well during the Depression. I love to garden, though I only have some small pots on my deck now. But one of my daughters lives on a farm and I go there to can fruit with her."

"You still can your own food?" I ask, finding it astonishing to envision this petite, still attractive 98-year-old, who resembles a slightly older version of Judi Dench, working over a hot stove with boiling fruit and arranging canning jars and lids.

"Oh yes, but now only applesauce, pears, and some jams like this apricot one. You just can't buy good canned fruit for one thing. It's not canned when the fruit is ripe." She takes a bite of salad.

"You're a calligrapher and a dancer, too?"

"I'm not a dancer anymore," Lucille laughs. "But I did love to dance. I enjoyed it so much that Sam, my late husband, had to learn. I gave it up after he had a stroke. But I still try to keep moving. I walk every day and do yoga twice a week."

She passes a bowl of fruit with fresh berries. "I am fortunate. Sam and I had a very successful and happy, long marriage. We were certainly distinct individuals and didn't always agree on everything, but we loved each other and were sensible enough to find ways to proceed. To begin with, our values, goals, and general natures were similar. It was a healthy relationship and I believe contributed to my longevity. I was very lucky, too, for my parents."

The food Lucille has prepared is delicious, and I am keen to learn more of her background.

"As I mentioned, my mother and father both grew up in the country," she replies to my question. "They had little opportunity for schooling. Dad had one year of high school and mother had only elementary school. In those days, farm children often had to move to town to get a high school education, and it wasn't possible for my mother. During the Depression, my father was unemployed for a long period. They both, however, were loving and excellent parents and made it clear they wanted me to have an education. I have always been curious and love to learn, and was the first in my family to go to college."

Lucille received a scholarship to Reed College in Portland. She took classes to become a medical technologist, and, while there, met Sam, also studying at Reed. They married while in college. With the advent of World War II, Sam postponed schooling to go into the forces, where he taught radar operation. After the war, he returned, finished school, and started a radio and television business.

"Before long we had four kids!" she says, "and I didn't remain a medical technologist for long. I went to work at Reed College, first at the bookstore, then at the admissions office, where I stayed for 20 years, until I retired. It was at Reed where I first became interested in calligraphy."

From the start, the art captivated her. Lloyd Reynolds was a professor at Reed College, where he taught creative writing, art history, and, for 20 years, calligraphy. I had heard stories of Lloyd Reynolds, and was aware that he had influenced many students during his tenure, including several who would become famous – Gary Snyder and Steve Jobs.

"It was a bit circuitous how I happened to take up calligraphy," explains Lucille. "I knew Lloyd for years. At the time when I was President of the PTA for my children, back in the 1960s, I asked him if he might do a class for parents. Lloyd graciously consented. He kindly let us use his own studio on the Reed campus."

"That's when you began calligraphy and never stopped."

"Not exactly. It was on and off at first. I was busy with work and raising children. I really got going after I retired. I discovered I loved it and began taking classes. I took classes once a week for 33 years."

"Thirty-three years?"

She nods, smiling at my unbelief. "I also go on calligraphy retreats, and have for years. I really enjoy them because I love the camaraderie. Until recently, I also loved to quilt and weave. I had a beautiful, big loom that I would work on. But when we downsized our home because Sam got sick, I had to give the loom away. I never, though, stopped doing calligraphy."

"That's why you are such an expert," I say, admiringly.

"Oh, not an expert," she quickly disagrees, "and please, I'm uncomfortable being called an artist. I have been a *student* of art," she smiles, "and always hope to get better. It keeps me motivated. My work is never perfect, but I love seeing progress."

That, I think, is the secret of mastery. Not to strive for flawlessness, but to endeavor to improve, which means we are all students. Cezanne, the famous French post-impressionist painter, is known for never stopping to try to improve on his work. Some of his best, most beloved pieces came late in his life.

"There are wonderful calligraphers in this city," says Lucille. "The people who are doing this art are active, interested in things. I have found, if you wish to have a long and satisfying life, you want to be surrounded by people like that. We all know people who retire with nothing to do and just sit at home. That's unfortunate. I love always learning something new! We only get one chance."

Lucille gets up from the table to put on the tea kettle. When she returns, she continues with her thought.

"A key is not to expect you can do what you were able to at 50 or 80," she says. "You learn to accept your limitations. You make modifications. The important thing: do what is possible and keep going."

"What is your secret for keeping going?" I ask, inspired by her vitality.

"It's quite simple, really. Keep moving! I believe, if you can walk, then walk! If you can play the piano, then play! If at all possible, stay mentally and physically active, and never, ever, lose your curiosity about life and the world around you. And don't be afraid to try new things. At 92, I took a wonderful trip to Vietnam with my daughter and son-in-law. I got to have my first ride on a motorcycle and was ferried across the city! I hung on for dear life, until I relaxed and saw how fun it was!"

She passes a basket of teas over to me. "Older people too often lose their confidence. They sit in a chair and quit trying. They grow discouraged, and think 'I'm on my way out, on my downhill,' and they just quit living. Sure, it can be hard. But the important thing is to keep trying at something that you care about and you will feel the difference. Be willing to work for something and keep at it. You get better at it. And I believe it is part of our human nature to want to be able to create something. I think doing art keeps people from giving up."

I remember how I lost my confidence after my accident. I *could* walk though, albeit awkwardly at first. What Lucille was saying made sense: just getting out and trying to do something was what brought me back. Not all at once, but in time.

Lucille's hazel eyes catch the afternoon sun and shine with youthful vigor as we finish lunch and take our tea with us to the living room to talk a bit more. On the table in front of the sofa is another merry arrangement of spring flowers – pink tulips, sky-blue hyacinths, pale yellow narcissus. On side tables, I notice works of calligraphy Lucille explains she is working on.

"There is always more to do," she says cheerfully, "and it keeps me challenged and absorbed. I know I am privileged to be here at 98, and blessed to be as healthy as I am. I was born into a loving family who made every effort to provide for my brother and me. I had good models; I chose a wonderful spouse. Not everyone has that. But individually we *do* have a choice in what paths we take. And we can always change direction if we will it.

"My family and friendships bring me the greatest joy. Seeing the next generations arriving is the most incredible gift. I have lost most of my older friends by now, but am fortunate to still have many younger ones through my associations. Just still being alive at 98 and able to experience more precious time on our beautiful earth is a gift."

Lucille places her china cup on the table before her. For a minute, regarding her kind face and nature, I find myself speechless.

"You need to understand, when you reach my age everyone will have suffered some sort of loss," she says, thoughtfully. "That is part of aging. I miss my husband of 65 years and I still can't talk about the death of my son, Greg, six years ago. Yet, while these losses are very real, there are others who still need me and whom I need and enjoy."

She startles. "Oh, the dessert!" she says, grinning. "I forgot all about it! I hope you like cookies."

"Do I like cookies? I love them!" We both start to laugh.

"Stay there; I will get them for us. Sugar may not be the best thing for our health, but laughter certainly is. One thing I think is quite important to a good long life is a sense of humor. It helps take us through all sorts of life's turns and twists, if we can nurture that. Laughter is good for the *soul*," says Lucille, rising from the couch. "We need to have fun together, first; then occasionally along life's path, the only solution is just to be able to laugh at yourself."

Smiling, still chuckling, she heads to the kitchen, where I can hear her arranging dessert on a plate. Spying a project lying on the table that Lucille mentioned she's working on for a friend, I pick it up.

It is a special poem, Lucille says, that a close acquaintance had asked her if she might hand letter in calligraphy. The book is to be a gift for her friend's daughter, a midwife who brings children into the world. Lucille, of course, takes the project on, adding that Psalm 139 is one of her own favorite sacred verses.

Studying it more closely, I encounter once more Lucille's remarkable script:

"O Lord, you have searched me and you know me.
  Where can I go from your Spirit?
  Where can I flee from your presence?
If I go up to the heavens, you are there.
If I make my bed in the depths, you are there.
If I rise on the wings of the dawn, if I settle on the far side of
  the sea,
  even there your hand will guide me.
  Your right hand will hold me fast.
The darkness will not be dark to you. The night will shine like
  the day,
  for darkness is as light to you.
I will praise you because I am fearfully and wonderfully made.
  Your works are wonderful."

Yes, I muse, they are wonderful indeed.
Dance, Lucille, Dance.

No matter what you do, plan! Make notes, look them
over once in a while, scratch them out when you finish
them, change them if need be, and try to be organized.
I have worked at things and not been successful.... I've
had major setbacks. But I never gave up. Each time,
I moved the track around a bit, reinvented it maybe,
searched for what was important to me, something
I believed in, and came back again.

Bob Moore,
age 91

7 THE GOLDEN SPURTLE

Marcy Cottrell Houle

The Golden Spurtle Trophy was something Bob Moore had hoped to win for years. And at 87, after months of dedicated work, his dream at last came true.

But what in heaven's name, I wondered, was a spurtle? Moreover, the significance of a golden one?

I was to find out, but not right away.

The sheer energy of the man sitting across from me at the table clearly is more than my own and, I rapidly fathom, could light up every bulb in the room. Now 91, this nonagenarian's dynamism and exuberance make me wonder if he might be an outlier on the map I am trying to make – perhaps more like a North Star that I can enjoy looking at and see shining, but never hope to reach. Bob tells me he still goes to work at 6.00 a.m. every day. He displays remarkable health and vigor, more than many half his age. On top of that, he has lived his life's purpose for nearly a half-century, and millions are benefiting from it.

What I know of his story is so extraordinary that, as he begins to relay it, I suspect that most people – certainly, I – would feel there wasn't much in it that we could apply to our own lives.

We would all be wrong.

Without a hint of stiffness, Bob leans forward in his chair and rubs his trimmed white beard, thinking for a moment about one of the questions I have posed to him.

"What gives my life meaning at age 91? Well, that meaning really hasn't changed much in the many years I've been living," he replies in a strong voice. "As to your other question, no, I have never retired. I do not want to retire! I love coming to work. I love people and being surrounded by them all day. I'm just as interested in building new machinery at 90 as I was at 30!"

I reflect, momentarily, about a study I had read in Tom Rath and Jim Harter's book *WellBeing*. In 1958, a research investigation conducted by George Gallup found that career well-being is one of the major differentiators that help people live into their 90s. People who had high career well-being awaken each day with something to look forward to doing. Bob certainly exhibited that. They also found that the sheer amount of time people spend engaged with others was a factor of good health and longevity. Bob obviously displayed that too.

"Making the decision to not retire and trying to plan for the future are two things that have been important in my life," he continues. "I believe no matter what you do, plan! Make notes, look them over once in a while, scratch them out when you finish them, change them if need be, and try to be organized. I have worked at things and not been successful. I've been broke twice. I've had major setbacks. But I never gave up. Each time, I moved the track around a bit, reinvented it maybe, searched for what was important to me, something I believed in, and came back again."

That track, a discernable trail of serpentine twists with scattered bursts of serendipity, would ultimately lead to great successes in Bob's life. For 60 years, he has been devoted to the idea of whole grains and healthy eating. In time, he would create a business – Bob's Red Mill Natural Foods – that today is America's premier whole grain food supplier, producing over 400 natural grain products with a worldwide distribution.

Like millions of others, I am a devotee of Bob's Red Mill products; just this morning, I had his organic oatmeal for breakfast. Elizabeth is also an enthusiast of Bob's – and she too follows the same credo: the critical importance of eating nuts, whole grains, vegetables, and fruits to keep your brain healthy.

"Years ago, when my wife Charlee and our three sons had our goat farm, we discovered a better way of eating. Charlee harvested fresh vegetables from our garden and gathered eggs from our chickens. She baked some of the best bread I've ever tasted in my life. Everything was organic. We dedicated ourselves to healthy things. From there, I started to plan. I had a vision."

"A vision?"

"To have my own business and operate my own flour mill."

I could not think of another person I knew whose vision was to have a flour mill. Intrigued now, I wondered how that became Bob's passion. He said his fervor to have his own business began early.

"When I was young, my dad and I would often stay up late, sometimes until midnight, just talking. My mother would come downstairs and tell us to come to bed, but many times we wouldn't. We'd talk about all sorts of things, like history, books, the importance of education, of politics. My father was in business for himself. He instilled that desire in me. Those conversations, and my growing interest in everything mechanical and in machinery, and my great love of music, formed me."

I had seen an upright piano when I entered the building, and another in the room next to the one we were in. I asked Bob about them.

"We have two pianos here at the company and I have pianos at home. When I was 9, I began playing violin and piano. I still play. Charlee learned too, and played well. We would play and sing together. And I play at the office ... every morning."

I smile at the image of the energetic, still amazingly fit man, dressed in his signature red vest, newsboy cap, bolo tie, serenading his employees. I glance around his office. Reading must also be a big part of his life. There are hundreds of books spilling from bookcases affixed to every wall. Favorites appear to be titles about food, aviation, archeology, biographies, and history.

"Learning has been very important to me," Bob says, catching me taking in the room. "It has opened doors of knowledge and has made me inquisitive. That curiosity has caused my mental faculties to never rest. I have loved to read my entire life. It is enriching and helps bring comfort during the hard times."

Bob admits there have been difficult transitions in his life, when all the plans he made didn't play out the way he hoped. He adds, though, that when that happens and life doesn't turn out the way you think you want, that's when you turn the page and make a new list.

Mentally, that was something I wanted to add to my map. Be willing to turn the page.

Bob tells me that his life has resulted in a number of new lists. He is candid about the ones that failed, and those that worked.

In 1953, when he married Charlee – his adored wife and partner of 65 years – Bob worked at US Electrical Motors. It was a job he loved – working closely with mechanics, electricians, maintenance workers, welders.

"That passion has never changed for me," he testifies. "Getting my hands dirty." In 1955, desiring to work for himself, Bob bought a Mobile Gas dealership in LA. While it was a great job and Charlee finally had her dream house, Bob hated LA and the smog. Together, they decided they wanted a cleaner, better life for themselves and their three young boys.

"We sold the house and the franchise, and moved to the mountains, where I purchased a Chevron station. Mammoth Lakes, a ski town in California, purportedly was on the cusp of becoming a major ski capital. Business would thrive! Unfortunately, Mother Nature interfered."

The season after Bob bought the business, the town of Mammoth Lakes experienced the biggest drought in decades – a winter of no snow.

"And in the scope of one year, we lost everything. Everything we had. All I had left was $450 in my pocket. It was a time when whatever could go wrong, did."

Needing to find work, the Moore family left the mountains and moved to Sacramento, where Bob found a job at an engineering and machine shop. With little money to spare, they needed a bargain place to live. One morning before work, Bob spied a small ad in the paper for a 5-acre goat farm available to rent. The goats and chickens went with the humble abode. They decided to take it.

That changed everything.

Having available space for the first time in their lives, Charlee planted a big garden. From the advice of "healthy eating cook books" by Adele Davis sent to her by her grandmother, she became converted to serving wholesome foods. Before long, she had transformed the family to a new way of eating. She even convinced Bob to quit smoking.

They thrived. Bob states that, by changing their lifestyles, they felt better, healthier, and were closer as a family. And there was something else. Inside Bob, a dream started taking shape. The outlines of it were vague at first. Then, in 1968, providence weighed in.

Frequenting the local library one evening, Bob picked up a book with a fascinating cover. At that moment, he did not know it would reinvent his life. *John Goffe's Mill* told the story of a man who, in 1938, left his position at Harvard's Peabody Museum to return to a family farm he had inherited. On it was an old family mill. What made the story so appealing to Bob were Goffe's descriptions of his work to restore the abandoned building and machinery. In resurrecting it, Goffe utilized what was, at the time, a lost art – employing old stone grinding mills to pulverize whole grains of wheat into flour. The result, he affirmed, was highly nutritious food that tasted much better than anything else available.

Bob had found his calling. The idea of John Goffe's mill combined all the things he loved – repairing motors and laboring with machinery – and the vision of a plan to help others achieve a healthy life. With the support of his family, in 1970 Bob purchased a building in Redding, California, that housed a small mill. With all their help, he got the mill running again, and in eight years the business, Moore's Flour Mill, was purring with success.

In 1978, the mill was smoothly taken over by two of his sons and Bob's dream was achieved. Nearly 50 years of age, Bob deliberated with Charlee that this might be a good time for them to both retire.

"And I did retire," he says, "for about six months. Charlee and I decided to pursue a different dream: to attend seminary at George Fox University, where we could audit classes. We made the move to Oregon."

"You transitioned from flour mill to seminary," I reply, amazed.

"That's not a big evolution. It's part of who I am. I have a deep respect for the Bible, and studying it has increased my determination to try to use it in my life. Reading it has created in me an interest in people and a sense of responsibility that we have to care for one another and for the earth. Seminary though," he clarifies, "didn't last too long."

Half a year after moving to Oregon, Bob was taking an evening stroll with Charlee – something they often did together – and turned down a rural lane. Before them, Bob spied a run-down, old mill sitting on what looked to be abandoned property. The deep-rooted vision stirred within him once more.

"I know people who say the best time of life is after you retire, but then all they do is mope around. I haven't lived that way one minute since I was born. From the moment I saw that mill, I knew I could never retire. So, we bought it."

Next, Bob was on the hunt to locate historic millstones. Successfully finding some beautiful specimens in a largely unpeopled part of the state, he bought them from a farmer and brought them home. Repairing them, developing new machinery, and hiring some help, he soon launched a new company that same year, calling it Bob's Red Mill.

"We had a terrific first six months," he says, "grinding whole grains into flours and cereals and growing our business. We were off to a great start and then, there was a fire. An arsonist burned down our mill. All that was left was the cement foundation. Once more in my life, I lost everything." He pauses. "After that, every-one expected I would retire for good."

But Bob did not. His employees stuck by him. Some of his product line was still unharmed. He had his clients. He sent whole grains to California, to his sons' mill, to grind and bring home. The business survived.

"We made it through. We rebuilt Bob's Red Mill, and we grew. Not only that, we became tremendously successful. In 2003, we opened our 'Whole Grain Store and Visitors Center' in Milwaukie, Oregon. In 2007, we moved our production headquarters to a larger facility.

"But, as I've seen in life, you can't take it with you," he con-tinues. "While everyone wishes for great success, there is a risk to it. For most people – and I am not immune – the allure of keeping profit and power for yourself can change you. It can change your values and how you relate to people. It is a fierce force – a battle that any reasonably successful person needs to fight. So, considering my age, I made a different decision."

Ten years ago, after careful deliberation and discussion with Charlee, Bob gave his company to the employees who had been there for him. With no strings attached, he created an employee-stock ownership plan for all who work for him, now totaling more than 600 people.

"I remain the President of the company. I still love to come to work every day. I am not retired! And," he laughs, "not everyone can say they are the recipient of the Golden Spurtle!" Smiling and ever amiable, Bob points to the unusual but handsome trophy proudly displayed on a table. It is easy to see why all the people who work for Bob love him. "I became the winner of the world's best porridge!"

Three years shy of 90, Bob entered the competition. After practicing at home for five months, he and Charlee travelled to Carrbridge, Scotland, to contend for the coveted honor. Numerous other competitors were there, all far younger than he, coming from all parts of the globe.

A spurtle, Bob explains, is a wooden kitchen tool that dates back to the fifteenth century. The implement resembles a cross between a paddle and a spear. For generations, spurtles have been used to stir soups and broths, stews and porridge. In Scotland, a spurtle is usually crafted from cherry wood or maple.

"I had my own made from myrtle wood – a beautiful, broadleaf evergreen tree found in Oregon."

"Did you have a secret, your winning strategy?"

"There is no secret. It is just good oats. We mill the best, most flavorful grains. Contestants, you see, bring their own oats with them. For the porridge, a contender is allowed to only have oats, water and salt. During the match, however, there is one potential but significant pitfall – intrusions. Organizers interrupt you, not on purpose of course, but they come over to pester you with questions, right when you are concentrating on timing and stirring. They stick a microphone in your face and ask you where you're from and quiz you. I practiced over and over, asking my employees to interfere with my concentration, so I would be prepared."

Bob won the "best porridge in the world" match hands-down. "It was a wonderful evening in Carrbridge that night," he says, grinning. "Carrbridge is a delightful, small Scottish village of about 750 people. The whole town came out. We went to a pub and were celebrated with bagpipes. Charlee and I never had a better time in our lives!

"I may be stubborn, but from my quiet, backwoods perspective, the best thing I have ever done is to keep working. My advice to others is, 'For Heaven's sake, do not let go of your job! Keep it!' I like helping others. I love the people I work with. They are my people. I am very pleased with my life. And Charlee would not want me to quit. She died six months ago, and I miss her terribly. She was my life's partner; the absence of her spirit is intense, especially at night, when I go home.

"She is with me, though. She is still with me," he says, in a softer tone. "After work, when I get home, and I feel lonely, I pour myself a glass of wine. Then, I go to my piano. I sit there for a moment and begin playing songs she loved and we would sing together."

A look of tender caring crosses Bob's face.

"I play for Charlee."

8 IS RETIREMENT BAD FOR MY HEALTH AND WELL-BEING?

Elizabeth Eckstrom, MD, MPH, MACP

Daniel Pink, in his book *Drive*, poses an intriguing thought. "At 60, people ask: 'When am I going to do something that matters? When am I going to live my best life? When am I going to make a difference in the world?'"

I love these questions. What they mean is that we all believe that at 60 we still have much to offer the world. Yet what does the world offer 60-somethings? *Retirement!* Which for some can be one of the biggest risk factors for death!

How in the world will anyone reach their full potential if all they do is retire?

One of our biggest failings in the US is the very notion of retirement. It causes us to lose tremendous human capital, not to mention loss of autonomy, mastery, and purpose. For many, the 50s and 60s are the most productive years of life. We have a wealth of experience; we don't suffer from the poor judgment or distractions of youth; we have strong communication and organizational skills. Yet many healthy, successful middle-aged people are actively planning for retirement ... to do what? Travel? Play golf? Learn to cook?

How many exotic trips, golf games, or new recipes does it take to get tired of this new life?

Trust me – far fewer than you anticipated.

Since so many of us are looking forward to retirement, it says something about the culture of work in America and our own experiences with it. "Work" for many is a four-letter word, better left unsaid. We are either in jobs that hold little passion or intellectual stimulation for us, and feel we are just "marking time," or we have an interesting job that hasn't changed over time and hasn't allowed us to meet our full potential.

When I was young, my father gave me some interesting advice. He said, "If you don't switch directions every seven years you will become bored. And you won't give the world all you have to offer."

While I haven't quite followed the seven-year rule, I certainly have found that making periodic major shifts in my professional life has led to opportunities for creativity and sharing that I could never have imagined.

Recognizing the loss of combined knowledge and experience that comes from retirement, and our own innate desires to live purposeful and creative lives, shouldn't we start early to make work meaningful, inspiring, and flexible over time, so we don't feel the urge to retire? Can we change the culture around work to consciously adapt to needs and desires of older workers?

Can we rename retirement "repurposing"?

More research is needed on strategies to assist older adults in finding a repurposed career that recognizes our need for autonomy, mastery, and purpose. We need to find approaches that attend to physical and cognitive changes that will occur. Many times, these modifications aren't too difficult to accommodate.

Let's start with the pluses of growing older. Older workers have experiential wisdom. They have continued enhancements to language skills; less need for financial remuneration; stronger commitments to family, community, and philanthropy; and a host of other positives. Who doesn't want to work side by side with people who have these skills?

At the same time, we also need to be practical about normal changes with aging (see Part II of this book). We might need shorter workdays to accommodate lessening energy levels, longer time periods to accomplish tasks due to reduction in speed of processing, and/or environmental changes to relieve arthritis pain or low vision.

Employers might feel they cannot afford these accommodations. Research shows, however, when real-life companies have made adjustments for older workers, and then offered these adjustments to younger workers too, the overall productivity of the company *increases*!

Even more interesting: Blue Zone regions – those five places in the world with the highest number of centenarians (people who have lived to be over 100) – don't have a retirement concept! People 90 and older continue to fish, to farm, and to care for children and grandchildren. They contribute meaningfully to society.

To learn more, watch the fascinating documentary *Coming of Age in Aging America.*

But back to my original question: Is retirement bad for your health and well-being? The results are actually mixed, and need to be individualized.

If your job is stressful and sedentary, it can lead to increased alcohol use, obesity, and other problems. Retiring from such a job may allow you to be more active, eat healthier food, decrease alcohol intake, and potentially add seven years to your life! In these cases, studies show that retiring can improve health, but *only* if post-retirement activities are purposeful, stimulating, and active.

Other studies, though, are not so promising.

A recent investigation in England showed that short-term memory declines 40% faster after retirement. Having had a cognitively stimulating job does not protect against this cognitive decline.

Another study showed that, after six years of complete retirement, people had a 5–16% worsening in mobility and ability to complete activities of daily living (such as bathing and dressing). Retirees also had a 5% increase in chronic medical conditions, and a 6–9% increase in mental health problems. These outcomes were thought due to declines in physical activity and social interactions. If the individual was married and had social support, continued to engage in physical activity post-retirement, or continued to work part-time upon retirement, these negative consequences of retirement are lessened.

There is more concerning data. Studies document that retirees are 40% more likely to have a heart attack or stroke than those who don't retire. The increase is more pronounced during the first year after retirement, and levels off after that.

For all these reasons, retirement is ranked Number 10 on the list of life's 43 most stressful events!

Another thing to consider is whether retirement is affordable for you. This is discussed in more detail in Part III, but it is worth noting that about 20% of Americans in their 40s have *no* retirement savings. Half of Americans won't be able to maintain their standard of living in retirement. Adults in other parts of the world appear to be able to plan better – as people in the United Kingdom save as much as 20% and people in China save as much as 50% toward their later years. If you want to retire, whether for health benefits or otherwise, you'll have to start preparing when you're still young.

Building new social relationships, making play part of life, finding new ways to contribute and learn are essential to successful aging. As Bob Moore shows us, making these things part of our ongoing work and for as long as possible, is a great way to be healthy and become your best future self.

All human beings deserve respect. The life of a general is no more important than that of a janitor. All are my brother, my sister, in humanity.

Yves Gineste,
founder of Humanitude

9 HUMANITUDE

Why Human Connection Is Vital for Everyone

Marcy Cottrell Houle

Too late. I realized I should not have accompanied John to his eye appointment. One week after my accident, yearning for a modicum of normalcy, I had asked to come. Admittedly, I did not look normal. With both arms in casts and black eyes extending down both cheeks, I resembled the boxer who'd lost the match. Yet, I reasoned, the opportunity to observe people going about their business would be a welcome change from lying on the couch, resting.

What I had not anticipated was the reaction of others when they saw me.

Actually, there was no reaction. People pretended not to see me at all, making a wide berth around my chair to select seats in the reception area far from mine.

With shock, for the first time in my life, I understood what it felt like to be invisible. People did not want to notice me – not knowing what to say, perhaps. But I had vanished from their view. In that moment, I grasped an awful truth: this must be how many older people feel, when they are ignored and isolated. For the recipient, faced with alienation, the message they hear is that they are no longer members of the human race.

My beloved father had disappeared from society when he developed Alzheimer Dementia. From being the highly respected physician he had been for most of his life, he became someone to be avoided, even among those who had been close friends. People are afraid of persons with dementia; seeing them kindles their worst fears about their own future.

I'd observed the same situation when visiting him at the nursing home where he recovered from a broken hip. Throughout the bleak corridors, patient room after patient room looked empty, except for the patients themselves, lying alone. Rarely would I see visitors. The patients had been erased from our view. Their lives were confined to a single building, their final chapters consisting only of scheduled pills and meal-times wearing dehumanizing pink bibs. With such terrible lack of relational communication, how could they recognize that they still had value?

All these people, and many, many more in our society, have – unintentionally or not – been labelled: "ceased to exist."

Now, months later and with my arms fully healed, I reflect on that experience while attending a conference Elizabeth has arranged. She has brought two colleagues to Oregon to lead sessions on the vital importance of human connections. Yves Gineste, from France, and Dr. Miwako Honda, a geriatrician from Tokyo, are teaching a program called "Humanitude" – a technique first developed 39 years ago by Yves and co-founder, Rosette Marescotti, and refined over 4 decades. Today, Humanitude is a worldwide network underpinned by years of research. It is being taught to doctors, nurses, health and care providers around the globe.

As I am learning, Humanitude is a methodology of care, through the exchange of looks, words, and touch, to provide well-being to those who have been estranged from society for reasons of age, vulnerability, or ill health. By being offered respect and compassion, frail elders are given value and dignity, and learn to feel they have not been abandoned. While primarily directed to those in medical settings, Humanitude is germane to all of us; people do not have to be sick or in the hospital to benefit.

Today in the United States, thousands of older people are living in social isolation. Elizabeth worries about numerous patients who are living alone. Research shows that loneliness leads to poor health outcomes. Social isolation significantly increases the risk of developing dementia and heart disease as one ages.

Isolation occurs in many ways. People can become alienated in care facilities, in the hospital, or even in their own homes or apartments. It is, Elizabeth says, a frightful feeling of being "written off" by others, of being disregarded by humanity. You become a ghost, and no one sees you.

Having experienced that scary feeling myself for 30 minutes was enough. It convinced me this would be an abysmal way to live out life. I was intrigued, therefore, how Humanitude might lessen such painful invisibility; and curious, too, to learn more about why Elizabeth is so excited over this new method of patient care and wishes to broaden awareness of this practice in the United States.

Earlier, Elizabeth had explained to me how she'd met Miwako and Yves. While on her sabbatical, researching places where people age the healthiest and best, her first stop on her tour was Japan. She visited hospitals, long-term care homes, clinics, patients' homes, and numerous communities. But what she'd observed at the Tokyo Medical Center rendered her amazed.

There, she encountered Yves and Miwako and got first-hand experience with the Humanitude caregiving technique. Never having heard of it before, she was curious to observe it, and quickly became enthralled by the approach.

Elizabeth watched Yves working with dementia patients at the hospital. He used kind, soft words to talk with them, offering a gentle touch and person-to-person gaze. Almost instantly, Elizabeth recognized improvement in patient eye contact and a reduction in their distress. Then, Elizabeth recounted a story of one patient he worked with. While describing it, her face held an expression of awe.

"As students in medical school, we learn about contractures," Elizabeth related. "I had observed patients early in my career whose arms and legs were stuck in a bent position, and doctors could do nothing to straighten them. When muscles or joints remain flexed for prolonged periods, you see, it causes them to become shorter and unable to stretch out. This limits mobility and function and can be very painful.

"The patient we visited was an older man in the hospital at the Tokyo Medical Center. His wife said her husband had suffered flexed arms and legs for more than a year. The man was staring blankly into space and occasionally moaning, presumably from pain," she continued. "I watched as Yves moved slowly over to him and with great warmth, gently touched him on the shoulder and gazed into the old man's eyes. When Yves spoke, his voice was respectful and tender. He continued this kind and loving communication for a few minutes, and then did something that took me by complete surprise.

"Very lightly, very gently, Yves stroked the man's arm for several minutes. Before long, the old man began to lengthen it out and straighten his arm. Then, Yves took the other arm. He stroked it the same gentle way, and it too became free. Yves next moved to the man's leg. Still talking compassionately and looking into the patient's eyes, he slowly stretched it out. The other leg was the most deformed and painful, but after several minutes of Yves' kind touch, the patient was finally able to partially straighten it."

"After a half hour," Elizabeth said, still with amazement, "and without any problem at all, Yves helped the man sit up! Now, instead of the vacant stare he previously had, he now looked expressively at his wife, and at Yves, and a smile broke out across his face.

"The man's wife was hardly able to speak. She was in tears," said Elizabeth. "She disclosed this was the first time her husband had been able to sit up, and, even more heart-rending, look meaningfully at her, for over a half a year."

That experience was what convinced Elizabeth that Humanitude training needed to be spread much more widely in the United States.

"When I returned from sabbatical, my dream was to bring Yves and Miwako here, to teach a program in Oregon," says Elizabeth. "I did just that."

Today's conference, the one Elizabeth arranged, is well attended by doctors, nurses, long-term care staff, and many others who care deeply about older adults. Like everyone else who learns about the technique of Humanitude, I find myself converted. The procedure employs practices of verticality (so many frail elders, Yves explains, spend all their time in bed!), blended with compassionate touch, speech, and gaze … and the results are profound. Viewing the training videos, we observe examples of patients who have been alienated from humanity appear to return to life. Some who have not stood up unassisted for months are able to rise and walk.

Patients who haven't spoken for long periods began to talk ... and even smile.

As Miwako and Yves explain, the basic premise of Humanitude is to teach us all *what it means to be human*. It is to help people who have felt alone and cast out to recognize themselves once again as part of humanity.

"All human beings deserve respect. The life of a general is no more important than that of a janitor. All are my brother, my sister, in humanity," Yves says.

At the close of the conference, I have the opportunity to visit with these miracle workers up close. Sitting at a table with Elizabeth, Miwako, and Yves, I remain fascinated to hear more about how they came to develop and put into service Humanitude, and learn what exciting new research is showing about its impressive results.

"We are *not* miracle workers," Yves quickly insists with a smile at me, "because what you see are not miracles! It's much more straightforward than that. What we teach is a simple yet profound truth: people are wired for human connection. Without it, they will die."

Yves' animated speech and tousled brown hair give proof to the liveliness that exudes from this Frenchman, the co-founder of the Humanitude program. He relates that the basis for Humanitude came about from what his wife, Rosette, and he both observed working together nearly four decades ago in a nursing facility in France.

"It was a terrible place – *terrible!* – like many hospitals at the time. They were much worse than they are today. Old patients lay crowded together in rooms, in inhumane conditions, and stayed there until they died. Each night after work, Rosette and I would come home and cry."

Driven to find better ways to work with patients, Yves and Rosette developed something they called the "tenderness touch." Using very soft and gentle movements, respectful communication, and an awareness of feedback, they began inventing and refining techniques that, in time, would change entire standard protocols for nursing in France.

Today, Humanitude is an internationally recognized network. With teams of over 100 instructors, practitioners have trained over

50,000 caregivers and health professionals around the world – in Europe, Africa, French Canada, and Japan. Yves and Miwako are now embarking on bringing this method of compassionate care to the United States.

"A baby learns he or she is human by love," explains Miwako, softly. "A mother's caress triggers activity that improves cognition and a baby's developing brain. Humans cannot develop without love and tenderness."

Miwako's gentle tone, serene composure, and youthful face add approachability to her sterling credentials. Trained first as a lawyer, Miwako relates that she developed a yearning to do something more to help people. She decided to switch careers, went back to medical school, and, after years of training, became a geriatrician. Miwako admits she discovered Humanitude by accident.

"I was traveling on a plane to attend a conference, and read about it in a magazine. I kept the magazine, and couldn't keep the story out of my mind. Some time later, I contacted Yves in France."

At his invitation, Miwako flew to Paris to participate in Humanitude training. Learning more, she knew this was something she wished to bring to her own practice of medicine. Before long, she was teaching it around the world.

"As a geriatrician, I work with many older patients," Miwako says. "Regardless of if they have ill health or dementia or are poor, everyone needs to feel respected and cared about in their communities. They need connection with others. A kind gaze, a gentle touch, or tender speech immediately triggers oxytocin, and releases in people confidence and love. Unfortunately," she adds, with a light frown, "too many seniors end up trapped in their own living arrangements and cannot get out into society. They become cut off socially . . . removed from humanity."

This is especially true for those in nursing homes, she explains. Miwako relates findings from a study of 100 bedridden persons with dementia in a care facility. In a 24-hour period, researchers found that patients were spoken to for only *2 minutes.*

"They may be dressed by aides and given pills, but this kind of forced care is not communicative," she says, with emotion. "To a defenseless person, what comes across is, 'If I don't look at you, if I don't talk to you, you do not exist. You live in isolation.' What we forget is how vital it is to reach out to others! Especially the old and vulnerable. A friendly smile, a kind word, a look at their face and into their eyes, validates them as a *person*, and lets them know they are not alone."

Studies of hundreds of patients in care settings where Humanitude is offered, Miwako shares, reveal a very different scenario – one which provides another reason Elizabeth is keen to bring this therapy to the United States. Nursing home facilities utilizing Humanitude procedures have been shown to *reduce the incidence of delirium, agitation, and the use of anti-psychotic drugs by as much as 88%.*

"Each time I look at you, each time I talk to you, I am speaking to your brain," says Yves, thoughtfully. "If I give you love and respect, I am letting you feel you belong to the human species. If I disregard you, it leads to your depersonalization. The most important thing in caring for others? It is tenderness."

I am touched by his words, making a note to include them on my map. Then, what he says next tickles me, since I live on a sheep farm.

"We all need to know who we are and how we belong," continues Yves. "A ewe, licking her newborn lamb, lets it know it is part of her species. She is putting it in 'lambitude'! We don't lick people, obviously, but we give them tenderness all the same. We want them to know *they are human*. We put them in *humanitude*. Emotional response, we know, comes before brain response."

I mull over this thought, thinking about how I communicated with my father as his Alzheimer Dementia progressed. Many times, he could not understand my words but he could always understand the love I had for him.

"The goal of Humanitude is not to 'cure' a person, but to 'care' a person," says Yves. "It is to love your brother and your sister. Even with persons with dementia, they may not *remember* you, but they can *feel* you. This all makes sense to me, of course. I'm French! I'm made for love!" he laughs.

May we all be French.

As she rises up from the table to depart, Miwako says something that suddenly touches the deepest part of my soul. Her words, and the sweetness of the way she says them, evoke a memory of the one thing we had hoped to give my beloved father throughout his Alzheimer Disease struggle, and especially during the last months of his life. In my heart, I like to think we succeeded.

"All people deserve to stay a citizen of humanity," says Miwako softly, "until their final day."

Your own joy increases when you make someone else happy. It's another way to make new friends ... Doing things for friends takes your mind off yourself. When you just think "poor me!" joy runs away from you.

Eleanore Rubenstein,
age 106

10 106 PROOF

Marcy Cottrell Houle

Eleanore Rubenstein comes to the door to welcome me into her home – a one-story ranch house with four large pots of colorful flowers at the entry. I have not seen her since before my accident, when we both were speakers at a Portland State University conference on aging and discussing themes from *The Gift of Caring*. That late fall day, Eleanore sat up front with me for a small panel discussion. Dressed in a timeless herringbone suit, her coiffed silver hair topped with a jaunty hat tilted at a fetching angle, her nails done, Eleanore was a sensation. Throughout the entire presentation, all eyes were only on her. She fielded dozens of questions, people wanting to know her secret.

I did too. You see, Eleanore is 106 years old.

"There is no secret," she says, straightforwardly, as she puts a kettle on to boil for tea. "That's why I couldn't answer their questions. I hope they weren't too disappointed."

"They weren't disappointed," I smile, catching sight of a framed quote hanging on the wall of her kitchen: *You are never too old to set a new goal or dream a new dream.* "That's lovely," I say, wondering if this is part of her secret.

"One of my grandchildren put that up," she says, bringing over a basketful of tea bags to choose from.

"So what are your goals? Your new dreams?"

"Don't have any." She selects English Breakfast. "Other than each day I am just glad to be alive." The phone rings. Eleanore lets the answering machine pick it up. "It's my son. He calls me every morning at 11:00. Then Dianne calls. She wants to know if I've taken my pills out of the pill box for the day. I don't take many, just one for high blood pressure and Vitamin D."

The phone rings again, right on schedule.

"Don't worry. I will call Dianne back. The others will be calling soon."

Not even noon, it is a bustling household.

"Thinking more about it, if there was a secret, which there isn't, it's probably a few things I've been blessed with. I'm lucky to have good health. Aside from having my tonsils and adenoids out when I was a child, and surgery for colon cancer, I've never been in the hospital. I keep busy. And I have a wonderful family."

I'm caught off guard for a moment. Colon cancer, of course, is a very serious illness. Eleanore, though, doesn't appear to see it that way any longer, which may in part explain why she is so robust now. She tells me she is the mother of four children, ranging in age from 76 to 85, and the grandmother and great-grandmother to many.

"I lost my husband when I was 67," she continues. "He was a clothing store owner and a good man. It's nice having someone live with you. But we are foolish to think that's not going to change. You learn to accept that." The phone rings again. "The answering machine will pick it up. I am grateful because I have wonderful friends and family. I think about the people who are so alone in the world that they don't have someone to call, to make them a cup of tea or a sandwich, or to take them somewhere. It is very sad. That's why it's important to keep making new friends. Many of your older friends will die."

Eleanore intones it so matter-of-factly that I am a little startled. "They die, and I go to their funerals," she continues. "I am very sorry to lose them, of course! But I keep meeting new people. My children's and grandchildren's friends are also mine, through them. They are all good to me. Instead of sitting around worrying, I keep myself busy. I love what I do."

"What do you do?" I asked, trying to imagine what kinds of things employ a busy centenarian's time.

"I volunteer. You'd be astonished how much your own joy increases when you make someone else happy. And it's another way to make new friends. I work at a place called "Start a Door," with other volunteers. I think volunteers as a whole are an unself-ish group, don't you? At "Start a Door" I phone people who are homebound and take orders for anything Kroger carries. Which is really everything but a car. We get their orders for drugs and food and diapers." She pauses. "Many are incontinent," she explains. "I pass along the list, and another person does the picking up and the third person does the delivery. It demands volunteers. And people are so grateful, you'd be surprised. Just so grateful for the help. Some people say it is lifesaving to them."

"Are these people shut-ins?" I ask, thinking about the danger of isolation. Of everything Yves and Miwako are trying to do. Of Humanitude. That is what Eleanore is offering to others.

"Yes, they are people who can't get out at all. And most don't seem to know anyone who can help them. There are a lot of people out there like that."

The phone rings again. Again, she does not answer it. Eleanore is right in what she is saying. In our current world, research is showing the sad fact that many people feel great loneliness, and it doesn't matter what their age is. While many may have dozens or hundreds of Facebook friends, the number of true friends people enjoy is decreasing. One highly concerning study concluded that 1 out of 10 people report they have no close friendships at all.

"So, you go to "Start a Door" and talk to these people on the phone," I continue.

"Yes. Every Tuesday. And sometimes I visit them. Last week a friend took me to the apartment of one of the ladies I talk to and wanted to meet. The lady is bedridden. She was so pleased to see me, and I her. It was wonderful. For I know how easily I could be on the receiving end of that. Really, it's a miracle that I'm not."

After our tea, we move to her living room. There are pictures of family displayed everywhere. "You still live alone?"

"I have lived in this house for 60 years. I do have a caregiver who checks in on me. She's done that for the last 19 years! She lives a few doors down. She is always ready to help me should I need it, and my children are happy to know she's there. Two of my daughters live only 5 to 10 minutes away. I see them all the time."

Clearly, Eleanore is not isolated. But I am still amazed that she lives independently and cares for herself.

"People around me are so good to me. I couldn't have got where I am without their help. And I know there's somebody up there looking down on me. Helping me. I'm a firm believer in that.

I think none of us really can run our lives without help. Every morning when I wake up I say 'thank you.' *Thank you, God, for another day. Another good day.*"

"Have you been this positive your whole life?"

"I think so, but probably without knowing it. And I think I've become more positive as I've gotten older."

"How is that? Because so many older people start to feel a little down or blue."

"Well, I think it's because I've always enjoyed life. I can't find any fault with my health. My children are wonderful. And I try to stay alert and active. I may not be able to play tennis anymore, which I loved. I had to give it up when I turned 92; my legs didn't like it. I can still golf, although my game more closely resembles croquet. People give up too early. You're not old at 65. I was just starting then. I can still knit. I can still play bridge. Do you play bridge?"

I shake my head.

"Bridge is good for your brain, you know. You should think about it. I've been playing bridge for as long as I can remember. Probably since the *Mayflower* arrived."

The phone rings again. I can't help asking how many phone calls she gets every day.

She pauses for a minute as if to add them up. "Oh, 12, 15 maybe. I get them in the morning and then again in the latter part of the day. It's my kids, daughters and sons-in-law, and grandchildren. And sometimes my dentist. He and his wife bring me over some meals, and we always have a cocktail."

I try to remember the last time I got 15 calls a day. Probably never.

"They are all trying to help me," she chuckles, "and, while I don't need it, I appreciate it. I don't think we were meant to live our lives without helping people. Plus, it gets you involved. I've always been involved. I find things to do.

"I've had friends of my daughters say to me 'but my mother never could do such and such!' I say, 'your mother never *liked* to do such and such. But she liked baking. She could bake cookies for someone.' Everybody has something they like and can do! And, whenever possible, make new friends. Doing things for friends takes your mind off yourself. When you just think 'poor me!' joy runs away from you."

It was an interesting verbal image ... Joy runs away from you when you focus just on yourself. It harked back to what Rabbi Stampfer elucidated – that if you set out to *find* happiness, happiness will elude you.

"Having friends is what makes life bearable," Eleanore continues. "Years ago, this became perfectly clear to me. I was in the hospital for some ailment. I was walking down the hall for a little change of scenery and a lady called out from her room, 'Will you take me to the bathroom?' I said 'Call the nurse.' She said, 'I have been. Nobody's come!' So I walked in her room.

"I saw she'd peed all over herself. I helped her sit up and then stand. I said to her, 'You have the most beautiful legs.' And she did! And she was not a young woman. She told me she'd danced with the San Francisco ballet for years. Never married, had no children, had nobody. I felt terrible. I don't know whatever happened to her. I can't imagine having no one. What an awful feeling it must be to be so alone."

Eleanore glances over at her phone.

"I better start calling back soon or they will be worrying about me. I know I am blessed to have someone worrying about me."

"I think you are, Eleanore."

"But you have to *do* something too," she adds, like an instruction I may have missed. "You have to think about making someone else happy."

There it was. Eleanore's secret. 106 Proof. Bringing joy to others, focusing on others, is the surest way to know joy yourself.

11 KILLING US QUIETLY
Why Social Isolation Is as Bad for Us as Smoking

Elizabeth Eckstrom, MD, MPH, MACP

Did you know that older adults who experience social isolation are at as high risk of dying as those who smoke 15 cigarettes daily or drink more than 6 alcoholic drinks per day?

I write this chapter at a time when we are all experiencing physical isolation during the COVID-19 pandemic. I bet every single one of us is suffering from the lack of connections! Notice I said we are all experiencing *physical* isolation. Many of us are really trying to stay socially connected – by calling family and friends (even some we haven't spoken with in years!) and using Zoom, FaceTime, and other platforms to see each other. We are also texting and writing letters (No kidding! How many of you did that for the first time in years?). We have learned more than ever how important personal connection is, and as the pandemic lessens its grip on the world, we gratefully eschew Zoom for real time together.

But a surprising number of older adults experience this type of isolation *every day*, even without the constraints of a pandemic. They have no one to connect with physically or virtually. Many of us may not realize that social isolation is truly another epidemic tearing through our society, with consequences for some that rival COVID-19.

Human beings are social creatures who thrive in collaborative groups. Our assemblages range from small family units to large college dorms. They include our schools, religious communities, neighborhoods, friends we go out with, and on-line chat groups. But as we age, those groups tend to become smaller in number.

Think about a young mother, who juggles childcare, school, and after-school events. She has a busy job and a tight-knit family. As her kids grow and leave for college, she thrives at work and in other social relationships, along with a deepening relationship with her partner (or maybe a new partner) and hopefully frequent visits from children and grandchildren.

When she retires, though, things change. Her partner possibly develops disability; she becomes the primary caregiver, with a much narrowed circle of friends and others she can rely on. Then her partner dies and long-neglected friends are no longer available to her. Her family might be far away and busy with lives of their own. Her world begins to close in. She looks forward to a weekly call from each daughter, and she goes out to the grocery store and to her hair salon, but has little else in the way of contact.

This is social isolation. It sneaks up on us over many years. At least one quarter of older adults in the US report feeling socially isolated. More people are living alone, fewer are married, volunteerism is decreasing, and fewer report a religious affiliation. All of these things lead to an increased risk of social isolation, with devastating consequences.

Social isolation is defined as someone living alone, having contact with friends and family less than once per month, and not belonging to some group (work, volunteer, religious, etc.). Men who are socially isolated (not married, fewer than six friends or relatives, no social groups) die of an accident or suicide at twice the rate of those not socially isolated. They have a far greater risk of heart attack and stroke. Both men and women who are socially isolated have higher rates of dementia and higher mortality overall, with doubled mortality rates in African Americans and 80% increased mortality rates in Caucasians.

Social determinants play a large role in whether we are at risk for social isolation. Our socioeconomic status, education, neighborhood and physical environment, employment, and social support networks, as well as access to healthcare, all contribute to its probability. Fortunately, health systems and insurance (e.g., Medicare in the US, the National Health Service in the UK) are starting to recognize the importance of alleviating the social determinants of health. Britain has a Minister for Loneliness, a Loneliness Awareness week, and a program to donate millions of pounds to small projects aimed at reducing loneliness. In some communities in the US, a socially isolated older adult may have access to a community health worker who can visit them once per week!

Social isolation and loneliness are *not* the same thing. Many people can be socially isolated without being lonely, and people can also be lonely without being socially isolated. We have very strong evidence, however, that both loneliness and social isolation are deleterious to our health.

Loneliness can be dangerous to health, causing depression, disability, impaired sleep, and other problems. Social isolation, while manifesting all the risks of loneliness, may have even more negative impacts on health. Additionally, if someone has functional impairment, memory loss, or depression from loneliness, they are more likely to become socially isolated.

What all this means is that we should be thinking about how to maintain *our own* social networks, and at the same time pay attention to *those around us* so we can help alleviate the social isolation of friends and neighbors.

Why does being socially isolated increase mortality? There are a number of theories. Social isolation may lead to depression, which also leads to increased mortality. Also, studies show lonely people express more inflammation because loneliness activates the fight-or-flight stress mechanism, which in turn leaves us more susceptible to inflammation and infection. Socially isolated people also lack contacts that may help them maintain healthier habits – for example, walking together.

Eleanore is lucky. At 106, she has friends and family checking on her frequently to prevent social isolation. But she also does many things herself! Her shopping assistance, phone calls to people she worries might be lonely, and simply waking up every day with a "thank you!" all help to reduce social isolation. Her volunteer activities force her to remain physically active, so she can continue to participate in life's important events.

What can you do? Here is a list of action items to help you prevent social isolation, or help you assist a family member or neighbor to reduce the threat of social isolation.

1   It sounds simple, but the basic goal is to *seek out social interactions*! Those who expand their number of friends have mortality rates that revert back to more average levels. Join a book club, become a museum docent, volunteer to read to children at the library. You may think you won't like doing these things, but if you stick with it, you will start to develop new relationships, keen interests, and feel renewed connections to life.

2   Reach out to cultural and ethnic groups that are unfamiliar to you. You will be surprised how this will reduce your implicit bias and you will discover new, rich relationships.

3   Take advantage of home-based healthcare, such as home physical therapy and occupational therapy. Look into home visits by volunteer organizations that provide home-delivered meals (e.g., Meals on Wheels). These regular visits can help reduce social isolation.

4   If you have ever owned a dog who needs a daily walk and plenty of attention, you will understand that pets can definitely help reduce social isolation.

5   Loneliness and social isolation can also lead to lack of self-worth. Maintaining a healthy self-image is very beneficial. But easier said than done! For someone who struggles with self-image, seeking out a psychologist for cognitive behavioral therapy can help.

6   Co-housing, where older people are living together or in intergenerational housing, can be a great remedy to social isolation (see Chapter 25). New, innovative housing communities are beginning to flourish across the US and worldwide. Tim Carpenter, one of my biggest heroes, started an arts-focused co-housing community called EngAGE in California. They produce their own plays and engage in many other amazing activities to encourage art and creativity in people of all ages. His vision has now spread

outside California – check out his website: https://engageda
ging.org.

7   The important thing to remember is *people need people*. No
matter what your age, it is worth the risk to reach out, to care
about, and to connect with others. It's what makes life worth
living.

12 BRAIN HEALTH ACROSS THE LIFESPAN

What Can I Do NOW to Prevent Dementia Later On?

Elizabeth Eckstrom, MD, MPH, MACP

Many of the patients I see in my practice are fit, engaged, productive, happy – in fact, terrific role models for healthy aging. And yet, they are afraid they are going to get dementia – or, worse, Alzheimer Disease (not realizing that Alzheimer Disease is simply one type of dementia). Even with all their successes – with loving relationships, meaningful work, and physical health – the specter of losing cognitive function is extremely troubling, and can even keep them from thoroughly enjoying their current health.

And for good reason. Many of us have watched our vibrant, engaged parents or friends develop dementia. Unfortunately, medical doctors can't promise that will not be the case for our patients or for their loved ones. There is still no cure for dementia.

But there is good news! Research shows life-long healthy habits may cut dementia risk by at least a third. The *Lancet* published a report in 2020 on dementia prevention, intervention, and care that shows some dementia risk factors (lower educational attainment in childhood, traumatic brain injury, etc.) are out of our current control, but there are many things we can do to modify our dementia risk in midlife and later (www.thelancet.com/article/S0140-6736(20)30367-6/fulltext). Employing healthy habits at age 50 reduces our risk for dementia for at least 24 years. And, even if you are already in your 60s, 70s, or 80s, making changes now will help reduce your risk of getting dementia. While up to half of people over 85 in the US suffer from cognitive impairment, people in the Blue Zones develop dementia at a 75% lower rate! Even more fascinating, doctors at the Loma Linda University Medical Center (located in one of the Blue Zones) believe that "If people truly live a healthy lifestyle, 90% should be able to avoid Alzheimer Disease within their normal lifespan."

Before launching into ways to protect our brains, it is important to understand what is considered *normal cognitive aging*, or how our cognition changes over time, even in the healthiest older people. Learning what is typical functioning allows us to discern whether we should be worried or not.

How Does Our Brain Change throughout Our Lifespan?

Throughout our lives, our brains undergo a process of gradual, ongoing, and highly variable modifications (see a detailed report on cognitive aging from the Institute of Medicine: www .nia.nih.gov/news/institute-medicine-releases-report-cognitive-aging). Communication within various parts of our central nervous system decreases a few milliseconds per year starting as young as age 20. The white matter in our brain – which connects everything together and transmits information – starts to decrease in size at about age 40, reducing "signal transmission" in the connecting lines. The retrieval and response times in some parts of the brain get slower. It is perfectly normal for people to notice slight cognitive changes by their 50s.

Scientists believe that what is going on is a phenomenon called "last in, first out." Brain areas last to develop in childhood produce thinner myelin – a protective covering that surrounds nerve fibers. A thinner myelin layer leaves these brain areas more susceptible to deterioration with aging.

The brain is divided into four main lobes: frontal, parietal, temporal, and occipital. Each lobe is "assigned" to different functions, and each has slightly different changes with aging.

The *occipital* brain lobe manages the perception and processing of visual information. It is the *first* to fully develop in the brain. Its function is generally preserved in healthy aging.

The *parietal lobe* is the part of the brain involved in sensory perception (awareness of touch, pressure, temperature, position, movement). It also develops early. These functions are generally preserved with healthy aging. It also controls our written and verbal language comprehension, which is mostly unaffected as we age.

Last to develop are the *frontal* and *temporal* areas of the brain. These lobes control memory, executive function and language. Being the final lobes to myelinate, they exhibit more risk for wear and tear. They are more likely to show decline as we age. Some decrease is perfectly normal.

Let's break this down a bit further so we may know what to expect.

Frontal lobes control our higher brain functioning. They are responsible for decision making, attentiveness, skill at multitasking, conceptual ability, and speech. In normal aging, we are still able to focus on one task at a time. But our ability to shift our attention between tasks efficiently becomes more difficult. This means that it gets harder and harder to double task – something we were probably never as good at as we thought we were in the first place! Slower word retrieval, name recall, and speed of speech is also normal as we get older.

The temporal lobe is important for memory and spatial navigation. Both of these functions diminish with normal aging. The volume of the hippocampus part of our brain, located in the temporal lobe, slowly declines after the age of 40. This causes diminished spatial navigation, which becomes noticeable after age 60 and further accelerated after age 70. What does this mean for us? It means we may have more trouble navigating, or finding our way in unfamiliar places, than we used to. For some healthy older adults, this can result in avoiding new environments and choosing to spend time in familiar places – which is just fine.

Memory is also housed in the temporal lobe. Everyone experiences some normal memory changes with aging. We have three kinds of memory – episodic memory, semantic memory, and physical memory. *Episodic memory* is our conscious recollection of events we experience. This declines the most with age. *Semantic memory* is our recall of facts, meanings, concepts, and rote knowledge and shows little age-related decline. *Physical memory*, such as guitar playing, playing the piano, or knitting, is the least affected with age.

Finally, normal aging also impacts our motor cortex and cerebellum. After the age of 70, our muscle strength decreases at a rate of 3% per year. The cerebellum loses nerve cells which leads to difficulties with coordination, slower processing and response times, and decreased gait speed.

How Does Our Biggest Fear – Dementia – Enter into the Framework of Aging?

First, let me give you some good news.

Just like the INCIDENCE of heart disease is going down, the INCIDENCE of dementia is *actually going down*!

What do we mean by incidence? Incidence is the percentage of a population who get a disease over time. Research is showing that *a smaller percentage of the older adult population is getting dementia.*

If this is so, you may ask, why does it seem every time I look around another friend is being diagnosed with dementia? That is because the PREVALENCE, or total number of persons with a disease, is going up. There are more older adults in the population than there have ever been. Therefore, even if there is a lower percentage of new persons with dementia, the overall number of people getting dementia is larger.

INCIDENCE, however, is a much more important statistic for each individual person. That's why we can take this as good news!

How Is Dementia Defined by Doctors and What Is the Difference between Dementia and Mild Cognitive Impairment?

"Dementia" is a general term for diseases that show abnormal loss of brain functioning. All are serious enough to impair social or occupational abilities, and interfere with being able to care for ourselves. Researchers who study dementia use the acronym ADRD – Alzheimer Disease and Related Dementias – to describe all of these cognitive disorders. Within this classification, there are four major types of dementia.

The most common type of dementia is *Alzheimer Disease*. This condition most strongly affects one's memory. It becomes increasingly challenging to learn new things and to remember events – so you forget what you had for breakfast, where you put your keys or glasses, and the name of someone you met recently. All this makes daily life frustrating. As Alzheimer Disease progresses, you begin to forget past events, lose language ability, and may develop mental health symptoms like paranoia, irritability, apathy, anxiety, and depression. Most people with mild Alzheimer Disease live about 10–15 years after they receive a diagnosis.

The second most common type of dementia is *Lewy Body Dementia*. People with Lewy Body Dementia don't have as much trouble with memory, but decision-making capacity is impaired, which makes it difficult to do finances or choose dinner from a menu. Also common can be visual hallucinations, sleep disturbance, and bad dreams. They may also have significant problems with gait and balance, and are sometimes mistaken for having Parkinson Disease, especially if they are early in their disease. Most people with Lewy Body Dementia live about 5–7 years after they receive a diagnosis.

Vascular dementia is a form of cognitive impairment that can happen after having a stroke or Transient Ischemic Attack (TIA). People with vascular dementia may have memory trouble, impaired decision making, language disturbance, changes in personality, and gait disorders. Most people with vascular dementia live another 5–7 years after their diagnosis, though this can be much shorter if they have another stroke or TIA. For this reason, doctors try very hard to manage vascular risk factors (high blood pressure, high cholesterol, etc.) in these patients.

Frontotemporal dementia is much rarer. It is characterized by major personality changes (often disinhibition), rapid decline in ability to care for oneself, and sometimes death at age 60 or even less. Most people with frontotemporal dementia live only 3–6 years after they are diagnosed with the disease. Dementia can also result from alcohol use (remember to stick with one drink per day or less if you are over 65), HIV disease, and other causes.

Dementia is not the same thing as *mild cognitive impairment*. Mild cognitive impairment means one has a decline in cognitive function from one's baseline, but it is not bad enough to cause impairment in daily function. As many as half of people with mild cognitive impairment could progress to dementia within 7 years. Luckily, up to 30% of people with mild cognitive impairment will go back to normal brain function rather than progressing to dementia, at least for a while – and living a healthy lifestyle is the best way to be in this group!

What *Can* (and SHOULD) We Do to Promote Healthy Brain Aging?

Good life-long habits can make a huge difference to keeping our brains healthy. They don't promise to prevent all dementia, but they are certainly *the* place to start! Doing them consistently makes you feel better, look better, and significantly reduces your risk of developing cognitive decline.

Research shows the following "Top Ten Practices" help to aid in keeping our brain healthy and high-functioning throughout our life.

1   Exercise, Exercise, Exercise

Exercise maintains or *even improves* cognitive function. In people with subjective memory complaints or mild cognitive impairment, moderate-intensity exercise improves cognitive scores. Several randomized studies of strength training showed improved executive function, particularly in women (and these effects are seen in people as young as 20!). Tai chi also has been shown to improve executive function, and the risks of tai chi are extremely low, even in somewhat fragile populations.

Why is tai chi so effective? It is thought to be due to several reasons. Tai chi is moderately aerobic (similar to brisk walking); it improves agility and mobility; it involves learning and memorization; it includes training in sustained attentional focus, shifting, and multitasking; it is meditative and relaxing; and even the social support of classes may enhance cognitive function.

Importantly, being active during non-work time at midlife has been shown to reduce the risk of cognitive decline later in life, so if you aren't currently active, *start now!*

2   Follow the Mediterranean Diet, or Eat Your Fruits and Vegetables

For women, having a Body Mass Index (BMI) over 30 in midlife increases dementia risk – so keeping your BMI in the healthy range is critical. The diet with the most positive research on its protective health effects is the Mediterranean diet. The Mediterranean diet improves cardiovascular health. More recently, this evidence has extended to cognitive health. People with the greatest adherence to a Mediterranean diet reduced risk of developing Alzheimer Disease by 33–40%.

The benefits from the Mediterranean diet in preserving brain health may be attributable to multiple factors. It reduces the risk of coronary disease, hypertension, diabetes, dyslipidemia, and metabolic syndrome – all of which are considered risk factors for cognitive impairment.

The Mediterranean diet focuses on fresh fruits and vegetables (try to get at least five colors per day – blueberries, tomatoes, squash, spinach, oranges …), whole grains, fish, healthy fats (olive oil, avocado, salmon, almonds, walnuts, etc.), and limit meat, dairy, and sugar.

(See Chapter 17.)

3   Participate in Cognitive Training/Stimulation, or Put On Your Dancing Shoes

A large study on cognitive training has shown some interesting results. The "Advanced Cognitive Training for Independent and Vital Elderly," or "ACTIVE" trial consisted of 4 training groups – memory, reasoning, speed of processing, and a no-contact control group. Over 10 years of follow-up, cognitive training was shown to slow both cognitive and functional decline. The speed of processing group experienced the biggest overall impact on health status.

What does this mean for us? Simply, a good goal is to learn something new every day! This can be learning a new language, or a new musical instrument. It can be learning a new dance step or a more advanced tai chi practice.

Pushing yourself to learn something new helps you *develop new neurons and new neural connections*. This is exciting news, indeed! By increasing your cognitive reserve, you can better cope with age-related brain changes.

4 Engage in Creative Pursuits

A study of healthy older adults engaging in creative activity (in this case, a chorale group) was shown to reduce doctor visits, medication use, falls, and led to better morale, less loneliness, and higher levels of activity. If creative activity is paired with social engagement, the results are even stronger!

This was demonstrated in one study that enrolled subjects into three groups. The first group used exercise plus musical accompaniment. The second used exercise alone. The third group was a control group, and did neither. The study found that the group who received exercise *and* music demonstrated more positive effects on cognition than either of the other groups.

Creativity, along with exercise and other experiences, helps increase brain plasticity, or neuroplasticity. The brain has a remarkable ability to reorganize itself, make new synaptic connections, and even create new neurons, or brain cells. Researchers used to think this only happened in childhood, but now it is clear that older adult brains also utilize plasticity to lay down new memories, recover from brain damage such as a stroke, and maybe even reduce the chance of cognitive impairment.

So, get out there and dance, learn a new musical instrument, and take that art class!

5 Sleep: You Need It

Inadequate sleep is linked to dementia and cognitive decline in older adults. Why is sleep of such value? Sleep helps remove beta-amyloid from the brain, which is the toxic compound thought to cause Alzheimer Disease. Seven hours of sleep per night is considered ideal for longevity. Normal sleep ranges from about 6 to 9 hours per night for older adults. But if you want to maximize your beta-amyloid clearance each night, try to get at least 7 hours of sleep. This needs to be done naturally since sleeping pills can cause dementia, falls, and other terrible outcomes.

6   Watch Your Medications

Medications are a major cause of cognitive decline. Sedative hypnotics, commonly called sleeping pills, are some of the worst. Drugs like alprazolam (Xanax®), zolpidem (Ambien® in the US, Stilnoct ® in the UK), lorazepam (Ativan®), and diphenhydramine (Benadryl® or Tylenol PM® in the US, Nytol Original® in the UK) should be *completely avoided after age 65*.

There are other types of medications that cause cognitive decline: drugs like cold remedies, bladder relaxants, muscle relaxants, bowel anti-spasmodics, and more. Unfortunately, many primary care providers are not aware these medications are so dangerous to older adults. Be sure to ask your doctor about potential cognitive side effects any time they prescribe a new medication, and check if the drug is on the Beers list (see *The Gift of Caring*, Appendix 1). The Beers list is a directory, as determined by the American Geriatric Society, of the drugs seniors should not be on but are too often prescribed.

7   It's Never Too Late to Go Back to School!

Another factor that can help reduce the risk of dementia is attaining a high education in youth. But taking classes may help improve brain function throughout life. Check to see if a community college or university near you offers free classes to those over 65. Many do.

8   Wear Hearing Aids

Uncorrected, low hearing has been repeatedly shown to lead to dementia. If you are hard of hearing, make sure to get and wear proper hearing aids. Correcting low hearing reduces risk for developing dementia. This becomes ever more important as we age. If you are prone to ear wax, get your ears cleaned regularly.

9 Watch Your Health: It Matters

As we age, it becomes even more important to be attentive to our underlying health conditions. Be cognizant if you have high blood pressure, obesity, or diabetes, and work to manage them. Following a good diet and participating in exercise practices, as described above, can make a big difference to our overall health, including our brain health. And be sure never to smoke.

10 Avoid Social Isolation and Recognize Depression

Social isolation is known to be a major contributor to brain decline (see Chapter 11). It is crucial as we age to get out into the community, and see and interact with people. Volunteering is a great way to meet those needs. Also, suffering from depression can affect brain health. Talk to your doctor if you constantly feel sad and unmotivated. There are very good treatments for depression that can be lifesaving and definitely help reduce cognitive impairment.

Some of you might say, "I may do all of these practices, but my parents both had Alzheimer Disease, so I'm sure I'm going to get it too!" Let me reassure you. A very large study looked at the impact of healthy lifestyle on dementia risk for people with low genetic risk and people with high genetic risk. Among older adults without cognitive impairment or dementia at the start of the study, a favorable lifestyle was associated with a lower risk of dementia *even among participants with high genetic risk.*

And for those of us who are women? A recent, very interesting study using PET scans (a type of imaging that shows function of an organ) showed "persistent metabolic youth in the aging female brain." In other words, the female brain has been shown on average to be about four years younger than the male brain. That is fortunate news for women.

While it's true that Alzheimer Disease and related dementias currently cannot be completely prevented, delaying their onset by even five years could reduce the cost to society by 50%. Engaging in a healthy lifestyle helps maintain our cognitive function and is valuable for people of all ages. The top ten habits, including exercise, healthy diet, cognitive stimulation, creative engagement, and healthy sleep, all help prevent cognitive decline. Too few older adults, however, practice these behaviors on a regular basis.

Let's change that! Take this opportunity NOW to think about your lifestyle practices. Add at least one new thing to your *dementia prevention regimen*. Keep up the "persistent metabolic youth" of your cognition. And celebrate a healthy aging brain.

PART II
Caring For Your Body

13 PROTECT YOUR BONES THROUGHOUT YOUR LIFE

Elizabeth Eckstrom, MD, MPH, MACP

From the time of birth until early adulthood, people build bones. This process lasts until you are in your 20s and sometimes 30s. How much bone you build depends on if you are getting enough calcium, vitamin D, and if you are engaging in weight-bearing exercise. After your 20s, most people will have a relatively stable bone mass for 10 or 20 more years.

That changes with age, more so for women than for men. Much of the alterations for women happen around menopause.

At menopause, women experience rapid bone loss for about 7 years. After that, women continue to lose bone, but at a slower rate. Some may take hormones during this time; these women do not have bone loss while on the hormones, but will have it when they stop taking the medication. Unfortunately, taking hormones is *not* the right answer to protecting our bones.

What is the ideal way to build strong bones? The answer is simple, straightforward, and natural. When you are young, the best things you can do are to run, jump, and play! Also, drink milk throughout childhood and young adulthood to get a healthy quantity of calcium and vitamin D. Doing this ensures good bone density when you get to the stage of bone loss. Encourage your children and grandchildren to get off their screens and get outside!

What if you don't have a great history of bone building? There are still things you can do, and should do, now and for the rest of your life to protect your bones. *Six lifestyle strategies* are essential to building a strong foundation for your body.

1   Exercise

To safeguard your bones and even build them at a later age, it is crucial that you participate in weight-bearing exercises. These are exercises that put force on bones, and include weight lifting, yoga, running, workouts with stretchy bands, and, yes, jumping jacks, because that old-fashioned PE drill jars our bones and makes them grow stronger!

Putting *force* on bones is the key to making them stronger. Bones only strengthen when they have some force on them telling them they need to be sturdier. Unfortunately, studies show that exercising in the water does nothing to strengthen bones because the water removes the force of gravity. Also, walking and cycling are not usually "jarring" enough to really help build bones either. They are great for our heart, but our bones just take a rest.

I recommend engaging in weight-bearing exercise for at least *30 minutes 3 times weekly*. Interestingly, our hip joints are tricky fellows to get to pay attention. Hips are positioned in a deep socket that has been built to protect them from harm. This is good, but it also means it is hard for them to have enough force applied to make them build bone. If our knees are okay, running downstairs works well and also jumping jacks will "jar" our hip joints awake enough to help build bone at your hips.

2   Bones Need Vitamin D

Vitamin D has an enormous amount of controversy associated with it, with research seeming to change on a daily basis. What is clear, though, is that bones do need vitamin D to strengthen them.

People used to get appropriate levels of vitamin D from the sun. Now that we do more work inside and have diminished ozone, we need to use sunscreen (SPF 50+) to protect us from the harmful effects of the sun. Sunscreen, however, impairs absorption of vitamin D, and increases the risk of vitamin D deficiency. *Please do not use this as an excuse to stop using sunscreen!* Sunscreen is vitally important to protect your skin from the harmful effects of sun exposure. What should you do instead?

The next best way to get vitamin D is through diet.

People need about 1000–2000 IU vitamin D3 (cholecalciferol) daily to protect their bones. Figuring this out is a case of simple addition. A cup of milk or low-fat, high-protein Greek yogurt contains 15% of your total daily intake. A 3-oz piece of salmon has over 400 IU vitamin – nearly half the recommended daily allowance!

For people who aren't milk drinkers or yogurt fans, figure out how much vitamin D you get from your diet on a daily basis, and then supplement the rest with a vitamin to get your minimum daily requirement. In general, if you get about one serving of dairy daily, I recommend taking about 600–800 IU cholecalciferol as a supplement.

3 Calcium Builds Strong Bones

Calcium also has controversy surrounding it but is essential to maintaining bone health. Ideally, the best way to get your calcium is from your diet. Dairy products are best, and contain 300 mg calcium per serving, but there are some other calcium sources such as seeds (poppy, sesame, and chia), sardines, beans (white beans are an excellent source of calcium), lentils, almonds, kale, edamame and tofu that can get you to your daily requirement without relying on dairy products. If you are not sure you are getting enough from your diet, a good number to keep in mind for calcium supplementation is 1000 mg daily.

4 Limit Alcohol and Tobacco

Both alcohol and tobacco use lead to bone loss. Quitting smoking is one of the best things people can do for themselves. Limiting alcohol intake to no more than one drink daily helps protect bones. People who have low bone density should consider stopping completely.

5 For Women, When You Are 65 Years Old, Get a Bone Density Test to Check for Osteoporosis

(Men don't need testing for osteoporosis until they are 80, and there isn't great evidence for it then, either.)

If the test results come back showing that you have osteoporosis, or you have a high FRAX score (a tool that predicts your risk of future fracture), it is worthwhile to take medication to build your bones. Of these medications, the most well known – and probably most feared – to build bones is alendronate, or Fosamax™. This is a highly effective drug. Many of my patients have averted fractures by taking alendronate or other medications in its class. Improvement happens within one to two years for many older adults, and I recommend taking it for five years and then reassessing whether it should be stopped.

So why are Fosamax and other bisphosphonates dreaded? This class of drugs has gotten a bad name due to stories of osteonecrosis of the jaw, a bone disease that occurs when there is a loss of blood to the jawbone. These problems are, however, far less common than we are led to believe, and usually related to IV bisphosphonates that are prescribed for cancer, not osteoporosis. I encourage people with osteoporosis or who have a FRAX score that predicts a greater than 3% risk of hip fracture over the next 10 years to carefully consider taking alendronate or another bone-building drug for a few years to improve their bone health. While taking the drug, it still remains critically important to make sure we get vitamin D and calcium, and, of course, continue weight-bearing exercise.

6 Prevent Falls: Falls Are a Leading Cause of Death in People over 65

While healthy bones will help prevent hip fractures and other serious bone breaks if you fall, the best way to protect our bones is to prevent falls from happening in the first place. Falls are the Number 1 injury-related cause of fatality for people over 65.

Falling usually has multiple causes, so it is important to determine all of your risk factors for falls, and then address as many of them as possible.

Many of the same strategies that help prevent bone loss also help prevent falls. Regular exercise is critical. Tai chi is the best exercise you can do to prevent falls. Research shows practicing tai chi can reduce the risk of falls by an astounding 60%! Making sure you get appropriate levels of vitamin D may help. Beyond these two recommendations, these three other evidence-based strategies reduce the chance of falling:

- Always wear the right glasses and footwear to protect from falls.
  Older persons who wear bifocals are at a higher risk of falling when they go outdoors. It is best to have two separate pairs of glasses, to be used for different activities. One pair should be for reading, and one for walking outside. Similarly, a good pair of walking shoes should be worn outside, and another sturdy pair of walking shoes should be at the entrance to change into for indoor use. The main thing: don't go barefoot or wear slippers or socks. Walking barefoot or wearing socks or slippers (aptly named – they make you slip!) can increase an older person's risk of falling tenfold!
- Make certain your medications don't put you at increased risk for falls.
  Check to see if your drug is noted in the Beers list, or "Drugs that Seniors Should Not Be Taking" (see *The Gift of Caring*, Appendix 1).
- Be sure your home is safe, and remove trip hazards and falling risks.
  Loose throw rugs, cords, dark corners, stairways without railings, poorly lit rooms, and many other common hazards in homes all increase the risk of falling. Complete a "home safety checklist" (www.cdc.gov/steadi/pdf/check_for_safety_bro chure-a.pdf) and make any necessary changes to make your home as safe as possible. If you have fallen or are at high risk for falling, have an occupational therapist come and help

ensure that your home is safe. *This is a covered Medicare benefit that your doctor can order for you.*

By paying careful attention to keeping your bones healthy, decreasing osteoporosis risks, and reducing the hazards of falling, you will greatly improve your chances of avoiding fractures. It's not perfect, as Marcy can attest! Falls and fractures do happen. But when you use these approaches to build your bones for a lifetime, you can help maintain your independence, which is worth every bit of the trouble of following all of these recommendations.

14 WHY YOUR BLADDER, KIDNEY, AND PERINEAL HEALTH MATTERS

Elizabeth Eckstrom, MD, MPH, MACP

Incontinence is one of the best ways to reduce our quality of life. Just think – if you are going out to lunch, taking a long hike in the woods, or sitting for two hours at a symphony performance, and in the back of your mind you are worrying that you might be incontinent, how completely can you enjoy yourself?

It is a very common concern. Many of us do have bladder leakage, or even loss of large amounts of urine, that bother us on a daily basis. If you are a woman and have had a couple of children, you are at even higher risk of developing incontinence later in life.

Starting *now* with strategies to improve bladder, kidney, and perineal health can truly preserve quality of life. In this chapter, I will discuss how you can maintain continence (a truly remarkable feat!), review tips to improving perineal health, and explain things you want to avoid in order to optimize your kidney function.

First, what does it mean to "maintain continence"? It can be defined as urinating only when sitting on a toilet or standing at a urinal, i.e., places where it is considered OK to urinate. This function, which sounds simple, is extremely complicated. To work, it requires efficient coordination between your brain, your spinal cord, and your bladder. The lower brain area, called the *pons*, has a "micturition center" – a collection of neuronal cell bodies – that helps us urinate when we need to. The higher brain areas ensure that we don't urinate when we shouldn't, i.e., anytime we are not sitting on a toilet.

There are also spinal reflex pathways that help to maintain continence. Diseases like stroke, diabetes, and spinal stenosis can disrupt these normal pathways. But even normal aging can cause disruptions. That doesn't mean, however, that incontinence is inevitable. It means *we need to be proactive in preventing it!*

Five excellent strategies can help decrease your chance of developing incontinence. They are also very effective if you are currently having trouble with incontinence.

1   Do Pelvic Floor Exercises 100 Times Daily

The best way to do them is as follows: sit on a toilet and begin to urinate. Then, try to stop your flow of urine. If you can stop the flow, this is a correct pelvic floor exercise. But please – never do this on the toilet again! If you do, you will train your bladder to not know when it is supposed to urinate! Doing it once on the toilet, though, ensures that you can do it correctly. This exercise is beneficial for women and men who lose urine when they are not sitting on a toilet.

Now, do this exercise 100 times daily when you are not on the toilet. Squeeze, hold for a second or two, and relax. You can do it anytime – while driving, watching TV, working at your computer, reading this book! You don't have to do them all at once, you can spread them throughout the day. Just be sure to get to 100 every day.

Research shows that doing this specific exercise helps many people become continent if they have bladder leakage, or at least leak less. Studies also show it works better than medications for many people.

If you can't stop the flow of urine when you try this on the toilet (and many women can't because they had children; many men can't, due to prostate problems), then I recommend seeing a physical therapist who specializes in incontinence. Physical therapists have lots of good ways to improve continence. And remember, pelvic floor exercises and pelvic physical therapy are not only for women – men have improvement in bladder symptoms with pelvic floor workouts too!

2   Do Timed Voiding and Drink Fluids

Have you ever sat for a while, and then stood up, realized you needed to go to the bathroom, and couldn't make it before losing a small or even large amount of urine? As we age, our bladders and brains don't talk to each other as well as they used to. We may not realize we need to urinate until our bladder is over-full, at which point we have no hope of getting to a bathroom in time.

The way to prevent this situation from happening is to urinate *before* letting your bladder over-fill. For most people, that means getting up and going to the bathroom every 2–3 hours or so – sometimes even more frequently.

Unfortunately, too many older adults don't drink enough fluid because they are afraid of incontinence. This can have dangerous ramifications. It can lead to dehydration.

Dehydration is exceedingly prevalent. It is one of Medicare's *top ten hospital admitting diagnoses* in the US. In older adults, it is the most common cause of fluid and electrolyte disorders. Dehydration can cause confusion, fatigue, low blood pressure, and falls, which can sometimes result in hip fracture. It is especially harmful in more frail seniors, becoming life-threatening rapidly and causing organ failure. The mortality rate for older adults suffering severe dehydration can be as high as 50%! Older people have diminished capacity to thermoregulate, and heat illness is common and can occur after just one hour of activity in the heat. Even more problematic, older individuals have a decreased awareness of thirst and often don't realize they are dehydrated.

The ability to recognize dehydration's early signs, therefore, can be critical. In early stages, an older person may only experience a dry or sticky mouth and dry skin. They may feel dizzy, have a headache, and feel muscle weakness. As dehydration progresses, dizziness may become more pronounced, which can lead to dangerous falls. Also, pulse rate becomes more rapid, and blood pressure drops. In severe cases, a person can become delirious or even unconscious.

That's why I recommend that everyone develop an awareness about the seriousness of dehydration! I recommend drinking a glass of water every hour, then going to the bathroom, and being active and moving for a few minutes. Drink a total of about 48 oz of fluid daily to prevent dehydration – more if you are exercising, outside in hot weather, or ill with a fever.

3   If You Have an Overactive Bladder, *Retrain* It!

Some people have the opposite of what I described above – rather than not realizing when they need to urinate, they feel like they need to urinate constantly. If you feel like you need to urinate very frequently – every 10 minutes or so – but then only dribble, don't despair. You can train your bladder to behave better. I tell my patients to try to hold their urine for successively longer periods – first for 15 minutes, then 20, then 30, and so forth. In time, this will retrain your bladder to not need to go so often.

4   Reduce Nighttime Urination

The need to urinate at night interrupts sleep for many people, regardless of age. This becomes especially apparent as you grow older; many older men and women need to get up several times per night to urinate. There are helpful things you can do to lessen this urge and protect your sleep.

- Be sure to drink 48 oz of fluid daily, but do it all before 6.00 p.m.
- Stop drinking fluids about 6.00 p.m. After that, just take sips of water with evening pills (if needed).
- Before bed, elevate your legs for 30 minutes, then urinate again, to help remove fluid that has built up during the day.

5   Avoid Alcohol and Caffeine as Much as Possible

Both alcohol and caffeine are bladder irritants. They can cause increased urinary frequency and urgency. For some, even one cup of coffee in the morning can cause problems all day and night.

It is also important to keep the other parts of the urinary and genital systems in good shape. These include the kidneys, vaginal area, and perineum – the region of the body between the pubic bone in the pelvis and tail bone. As we age, there is a slow but steady decline in kidney function that is inevitable. It is essential, therefore, to do everything possible to minimize that decrease.

How do you do that? Two methods are known to be especially effective.

- Drinking enough fluid – at least 48 oz non-caffeinated, non-sugary, non-alcoholic fluid daily – is critical to promoting good kidney function.
- Avoiding drugs, or decreasing doses of drugs, that are hard on the kidneys is vital too. Many people have heard acetaminophen (Tylenol® in the US, paracetamol in the UK) is hard on kidneys, but kidney problems with acetaminophen are actually very rare. It is definitely a safer pain medication for your kidneys than other pain medications. Anti-inflammatory drugs like ibuprofen (Advil® in the US or Nurofen® in the UK) and naproxen (Aleve® in the US or Naprosyn® in the UK) can cause kidney problems, and should be used cautiously or not at all in older people (especially if you also have high blood pressure, GI bleeding, or congestive heart failure). Prescription pain medications like oxycodone also can lead to kidney problems – so to be as safe as possible, stick with topical remedies like a lidocaine patch or diclofenac gel and use acetaminophen if needed.

The good news is that most older adults with gradually worsening kidney function *never* need to start dialysis. Most older people die "with" poor kidney function, not "of" poor kidney function (this is not true if you have developed poor kidney function at a young age, when the chance that you will need dialysis is much higher).

Also important for women in protecting your bladder and kidneys is to maintain your vaginal and perineal health. Thinning of the vaginal mucosa, or "atrophic vaginitis," can increase risk of incontinence and urinary tract infections. One of the best ways to keep the vaginal mucosa healthy is to have sexual intercourse. Many women have good reasons for not being sexually active, but if you have a partner and would like to be sexually active, I tell my patients, do it. It will reduce dryness and promote healthy vaginal tissue. If it is painful, speak with your doctor about ways to reduce pain with intercourse. Another option to reduce vaginal atrophy and its consequences is to use vaginal estrogen cream, which can be prescribed by your doctor. It is safe even for most people who cannot take oral estrogen. Be sure to talk with your primary care provider about this if it is something that affects you. For women who don't have a sexual partner, using sex toys such as vibrators may provide benefit too.

Many older people also suffer from urinary tract infections (UTIs). These are also not an inevitable part of aging, and we should do all we can to prevent them. The best way to reduce risk of UTIs is to drink adequate fluids. If you have vaginal atrophy, using vaginal estrogen may also help you reduce your chance of getting UTIs. Other prevention options – such as cranberry juice, probiotics, and D-mannose – have not been proven effective in preventing UTIs. They may, however, be effective for some individuals and are generally safe. If you want to try these products, I recommend doing it regularly for a couple of months to see whether it makes a difference. If not, then it is probably not worth the cost for you.

As with most of our major organs and body functioning, the urinary and genital systems go through significant changes with aging. Understanding what they are and planning for them, paying good attention to your fluid intake, faithfully doing your pelvic floor exercises, and following the other listed suggestions, can reap positive benefits that work well into very old age.

15 MAINTAINING YOUR BLOOD (CARDIOVASCULAR) SYSTEM

Elizabeth Eckstrom, MD, MPH, MACP

More than nearly any other organ system in the body, our blood system undergoes some of the most complex changes of aging across the lifespan. This system, also known as the cardiovascular system, includes our heart and blood vessels. Unlike dementia, urinary incontinence, and other potentially preventable aging problems, the changes that happen to our blood system happen to everyone.

Three features in particular undergo modification in our blood system as we grow older: our *blood pressure*, our *heart's pumping ability and changes to heart valves*, and our *cholesterol*. All three play strong roles, and in this chapter, I will discuss those changes you can expect. Just as we have seen with our other organ systems, there are ways we can lessen aging's impacts. Even better, as I will explain, research shows that as much as 70% of heart disease can be prevented or delayed with a healthy lifestyle.

Let's take them one by one and dive in!

Blood Pressure

You probably remember that when you were young your doctor always told you your blood pressure was about 120/80, or maybe even less. Now when you go to the doctor, they might say "your blood pressure is all the way up to 148/90. I am afraid we need to do something about that ... "

The reality is, gradually rising blood pressure is a normal change with aging. Our blood vessels become more stiff and narrowed due to accumulation of lipid (fat) deposits on the insides of the walls (more about this later). Our arteries change throughout our life.

Let's visualize a young person's arteries for a moment. They resemble a long thin balloon. The balloon readily expands and contracts as you add or remove air. For an older person, though, it's different.

As we age, that supple balloon turns into an iron pipe. It becomes thick, hard, and without much ability to expand or contract. That inflexibility in our arteries makes all the difference in regulating our blood pressure.

When you hear the words "blood pressure," what do they mean? What are those numbers – top and bottom – that go with it?

The top number is *systolic* blood pressure. It is the pressure that pushes blood *out of the heart* and into every corner of your body.

The bottom number is *diastolic* blood pressure. It is the pressure your blood exerts before the heart contracts, or while the heart is *resting between beats.*

Typically, the top number is a better predictor of heart health and risk of death, so we will focus on that number.

Now let's look at what happens as we age.

Our blood pressure changes with the activities we are doing. When we are young and exercising, our lithe arteries easily expand, lowering the pressure we exert on them while our blood moves freely to oxygenate our brain. Also when young, our arteries more easily contract to raise our blood pressure when we go from sitting (when most of our blood volume is in our legs) to standing up, pushing blood to our brain, which needs oxygen.

Once we have "iron pipes" for arteries, however, we don't have that same ability to regulate our blood pressure. Our arteries don't expand or contract as well or as readily. That first number? Systolic blood pressure? It elevates, because it's harder to push blood through those narrow, stiff arteries. (Voila! That's the reason for higher blood pressure!). And when we stand up, that pipe can't suddenly contract as it used to. So, the blood stays in our legs for a few minutes too long. We lack blood to our brain, and we feel dizzy, lightheaded, and unsteady. This condition is called *orthostatic hypotension* and is very common in older people. It can lead to falls, passing out, and other terrible outcomes.

If you are relatively healthy and want to live as long as possible, doctors may recommend a *systolic blood pressure less than 120–130*, whereas if you are older and frail and your goal is comfort rather than living longer, they may recommend a *systolic blood pressure of 130–140*. In other words, it is okay if your systolic blood pressure runs slightly higher, because the goal is quality of life over duration of life. If your systolic blood pressure is higher than desired, they may recommend taking a blood pressure medication.

I always encourage doctors to check *orthostatic blood pressures*, which is a comparison of your blood pressure when you go from lying down to standing, to look for drops in pressure. This is done by having the patient lie down for 5 minutes, and getting a reading, and then having them stand up for 1 minute, and getting another reading. These readings are important. If an older person's systolic blood pressure (top number) drops more than 20 points with standing, then it *may not be safe to get their sitting blood pressure down to 120*. In these cases, if they stand up too fast, there is not enough oxygen pumped to their brain and they can get dizzy and faint.

Sometimes people have higher blood pressure at their doctor's office. This is called "white coat hypertension," and is often the result of being nervous at the doctor's office. It does not necessarily mean that you have chronic hypertension, just that your anxiety (even if you don't recognize it yourself as anxiety) is causing your blood pressure to increase for the time span that you are anxious. If your blood pressure is high in the doctor's office but lower when you check it at a pharmacy or at home, it is a good idea to get a blood pressure cuff and check your blood pressure at home to share readings with your doctor.

Before adding any pills to bring down blood pressure, I recommend to my patients to try *lifestyle modifications first*. Surprisingly, simple things can make a big difference! Losing weight lowers blood pressure by about 1 point per kilogram, so if you lose 10 pounds your blood

Table 15.1 Interventions for reducing systolic blood pressure

Intervention	Effect on blood pressure
Weight loss	1 unit reduction in blood pressure per kg body weight loss
DASH diet	11 units reduction in blood pressure
Limiting dietary sodium to ½ tsp per day	5–6 units reduction in blood pressure
Brisk walk for 90–150 min a week	5–8 units reduction in blood pressure

pressure will come down almost 5 points! Following a Mediterranean diet (see Chapter 17) or DASH diet (similar to Mediterranean, but lower salt and a little more white meat and dairy) lowers blood pressure 11 points. Reducing sodium to 1/2 tsp per day lowers blood pressure about 5 points. A combination of aerobic and strength training exercise lowers it about 9 points (brisk walking for 30 minutes 5 days per week plus yoga, weights, or stretchy bands). Decreasing alcohol to 1 drink per day lowers blood pressure 5 points. Stopping smoking lowers it at least 5 points (Table 15.1).

What this means is, if you do all of those things, your blood pressure will be as much as *40 points lower* – which will almost certainly allow you to skip the blood pressure pill!

People often ask me which blood pressure pills are safe for older adults. There are several I turn to regularly (Table 15.2). Just be sure that, before starting any of these drugs, your doctor checks your orthostatic blood pressures!

How Does Age Change Our Heart's Pumping Ability and Our Heart Valves?

As we age, our heart may decrease in size a little. The wall of the left ventricle (the chamber of our heart which receives blood and pumps it into the circulation system through the aorta) thickens. This means the heart holds less blood. At the same time, the heart tends to fill more slowly. Also, the heart has a slightly slower rate

Table 15.2 Good blood pressure medications for older adults

Drug name	How it works	Why it is good	Side effects to watch for
Amlodipine	Calcium Channel Blocker – powerful BP reducer, so start with just 2.5 mg, can gradually increase to 10 mg if needed	Decreases heart risk, low risk of orthostatic hypotension	Leg swelling
Hydrochlorothiazide (HCTZ)	Diuretic (water pill), dose is 12.5 mg	Decreases heart risk	Frequent urination, orthostatic hypotension
Lisinopril and losartan	Works on the kidneys, start with 2.5 mg and work up to 40 mg if needed (Lisinopril); start with 25 mg and work up to 100 mg if needed (Losartan)	Protects kidneys, especially with diabetes	High potassium, cough

of pumping with age due to scar tissue that can build up in the tracts that control the heart's electrical system.

Another trend: lipofuscin, or "aging pigment," gets deposited in our hearts. These brownish-yellow fatty pigments are found in various tissue cells and are associated with aging. At the same time, the muscle cells of our heart decline. In addition, our heart valves themselves become stiffer and thickened. All of these things make the work of the heart harder and more prone to "fail," or not fully oxygenate our body for all the things we want to do.

And if you have confining, inflexible blood vessels with fat deposits on them? This condition is *atherosclerosis* – one of the main reasons people have heart attacks, heart failure, strokes, and peripheral vascular disease (a disease in which arteries narrow due to plaques). If the arteries in the heart have atherosclerosis, they can form a clot, which then causes the area beyond the clot to have low oxygen and die. That is called myocardial ischemia, or a term we all know – a heart attack.

Heart valves can also be problematic as we age. A heart valve is like a spigot that opens or closes a faucet. When open, the valve allows blood to flow in one direction through the heart. When working properly, heart valves allow only one-way traffic – they permit blood to move only in one direction through the heart. As we age, our heart valves do not work the way they should, making sure blood is flowing freely in a *forward direction*. Their performance declines and the faucet leaks.

With the heart's decreased pumping ability, flagging valves, and clogged arteries, you can understand why cardiovascular disease accounts for almost 50% of all deaths in industrialized nations (non-industrialized nations tend to fare better, as their diets and lifestyle better promote heart health and physical activity).

Cholesterol

Now we come to something that confuses many of us when we think about blood: cholesterol! A build-up of cholesterol within the arteries in our heart and throughout our body stiffens our blood vessels and lays down fat deposits within their walls (atherosclerosis, described above). We also know that high cholesterol increases our risk for heart attacks, strokes, and other bad outcomes. This is especially true if our "bad cholesterol" – LDL – is high, and our "good cholesterol" – HDL – is low.

But with all this knowledge, it is still tricky to manage cholesterol in people over 75!

For those who haven't reached that magic age yet, a healthy lifestyle remains paramount in decreasing your risk of developing atherosclerosis. If your blood tests for cholesterol are high, your doctor may prescribe a medication to reduce cholesterol. And, at *any* age, if you have had a heart attack, stroke, or peripheral vascular disease (such as carotid artery narrowing), you need to take a medication to reduce cholesterol (usually a statin).

But what if you have no known heart disease and you are over 75?

Here is the good news. If you are 75 years or older, there is *no clear evidence* that starting or continuing to take cholesterol medication helps prevent heart attacks, strokes, or other bad events. Wow! This finding also holds true for people who have a life expectancy of less than 10 years for other reasons (such as cancer). In all these cases, I still encourage you to keep up your healthy lifestyle, but more likely than not there isn't a good reason for a cholesterol medication.

While many things change about our blood system as part of normal aging, that does not mean we can't modify our outcomes. Major threats to our heart health – sedentary lifestyles, western-style diets (high in red meat and fat), cigarette smoking, and obesity – are major contributors to heart problems. But we know there are steps we can take that can ameliorate these risks, and make our cardiovascular system the best it can possibly be.

Five actions, in particular, are guardians of your blood and heart.

1   If you are overweight, work with your healthcare provider (or others) to lose those extra pounds. Excess weight gain and

obesity are known major risk factors for cardiovascular disease.

2 If you are a smoker, stop now!

3 Watch your diet! The best thing you can do for your blood system is to eat well with plenty of fruits and vegetables and omega-3s (think fish oil), and follow the Mediterranean diet (Chapter 17).

4 If you have high cholesterol, high blood pressure, or diabetes, work with your doctor to manage these conditions.

5 Lastly, you've heard me say this again and again: *exercise*. Physical inactivity is associated with at least a *twofold increase in the risk for a heart attack*. Exercise will absolutely improve your heart health.

Remember, as much as 70% of cardiovascular disease can be prevented or delayed. By developing an awareness of how the cardiovascular system changes over time, and employing ways to improve its function, you can enjoy more years of quality of life. What's more, your heart will love you.

16 OUR MUSCLES THROUGHOUT THE LIFESPAN

Build Resilience Now to Prevent Frailty Later

Elizabeth Eckstrom, MD, MPH, MACP

I heard a saying years ago that has stuck with me: "You think that extra weight you have put on since high school is muscle?" This question was meant to heighten our awareness about the weight gain that is so common in middle age, but it reveals something at a deeper level. Most of us *don't* build muscle mass after young adulthood. And this can cause a host of problems for us later.

On average, after we turn 50, our muscle mass decreases 1–2% per year. In fact, from our 20s until the age of 80, our muscle mass decreases by 30–50%. For most people, this becomes increasingly noticeable after age 70.

With the decrease in muscle mass, our strength declines by 10% to 15% per decade up to about age 70 – when this loss *accelerates to 25% to 40% per decade*. Yikes! With this reduction of muscle mass and strength, our level of general conditioning plummets. Without specific effort, older adults will continue into a spiral of deconditioning.

Muscle loss, or "sarcopenia," often serves as a harbinger of frailty. Many of us hold the belief that aging is a process of gradually descending into frailty until we can't care for ourselves or live independently. But this is not necessarily true. Frailty is *not normal* with aging. But there are many factors that can lead older people to become frail. Some of the causes of frailty are medical conditions such as heart and lung disease, lack of adequate social support, falls and injuries, too many pills, and being sedentary (not exercising enough). Three of the following five factors must be met for a person to be considered frail:

- unintentional weight loss
- exhaustion
- muscle weakness
- slowness in walking
- low levels of activity

These factors are not always the result of a specific disease – rather, they often develop from the cumulative effects of a person's socio-economic setting, lifestyle, and physical well-being. This is important because medical problems that are trivial for healthy people, such as a cough or urinary tract infection, could become unre-coverable events for people who are very frail.

One of the amazing people I had the opportunity to visit on my sabbatical was Dr. Ken Rockwood at Dalhousie University in Nova Scotia. Dr. Rockwood has taken a slightly different approach to thinking about frailty. He defines it as an "accumulation of def-icits," instead of by specific symptoms. He developed the "Clinical Frailty Score," which grades people from Very Fit ("People who are robust, active, energetic and motivated. These people commonly exercise regularly. They are among the fittest for their age") to Very Severely Frail ("Completely dependent, approaching the end of life. Typically, they could not recover even from a minor ill-ness"). The Clinical Frailty Score combines symptoms, signs, dis-eases, and disabilities (deficits) to come up with a score that helps to *predict a person's vulnerability.*

The Clinical Frailty Score considers all the reasons why some-one might have symptoms of frailty, but goes beyond that index to measure frailty in a very practical way. It includes what is still possible for a person *to do.* It is a tremendously valuable approach because it recognizes the complexity of an individual patient, and *helps to plan for future stressors in a person-centered way.*

The following statement is so important that I will say it again: Frailty is *not* a necessary outcome of old age! Rather, it is a group of symptoms that can be effectively *avoided* or *treated*. Among people over 65, 7–16% living in the community are frail, and by age 85 that number jumps to 25%. Look at those numbers more closely. They mean that most older people are not frail! Younger people can encourage our older family members and friends to improve their fitness, and keep up our own fitness level to prevent frailty when we are older.

Multiple studies have shown that a good exercise program, including aerobic, strength, and balance regimens, preserves muscle mass in older generations. So much so that the muscle mass of an octogenarian could *surpass* that of a 20-year-old! Engaging in athletic activity, especially resistance training, has been shown to decrease sarcopenia and thus prevent the first step toward becoming frail. Simply lifting light weights has been shown to increase functional physical capacity and increase muscle mass in older adults. Resistance exercise has been shown to improve strength and muscle mass even in people in their 90s! Practicing yoga, or using resistance bands, will also help prevent or reduce sarcopenia and help stem the ill effects of frailty.

A diet rich in omega-3 fatty acids, creatine (think fish such as herring and salmon, poultry, and occasional red meat), and vitamin D has also been shown to decrease loss of muscle mass. Adequate intake of protein – the building blocks of our muscles – is beneficial as well.

Older adults should get 0.7–1 grams of protein per kilogram of body weight, so an average-size older woman probably needs to eat 60–70 grams of protein daily. That is the equivalent of one large chicken breast, one half can of tuna, one cup of high protein Greek yogurt, and ¼ cup chickpeas, all in one day. But many older people eat far less protein than this. And for someone who has sarcopenia, they should be eating 2.2 grams of protein per kilogram of body weight!

It may be hard to imagine eating 2 chicken breasts, one can of tuna, 2 cups of high protein Greek yogurt, and ½ cup of chickpeas in a day. It is a real challenge to get this much protein in our diet, but it is critical to reducing sarcopenia, frailty, and loss of independence. Once again, the Mediterranean diet is a perfect choice to reduce frailty (see Chapter 17) – it reduces new-onset frailty by as much as 70%!

Another defense mechanism against frailty is the concept of *resilience*. This is a process of recovering from a significant stress, trauma, or illness, and returning to a previous state of health. Resilience does not come inside a pill. Instead, it is a *mindset* that is the result of many years of a manageable amount of stress that facilitates growth.

As patients, we often expect cures to be neatly packaged and handed to us by doctors or pharmacists, but resilience is not as easily obtained. Not only does it include persistent determination, but also the ability to seek out help when needed. Resilience is not simply an abstract encouraging notion. It is a studied mechanism proven to allow people to recover from frailty. It is not a concept specific to older people but something we should be building at all ages.

The stressors we go through – such as medical illness, problems with relationships and loss of family members, school failures or loss of a job, or even a pandemic – can all help build our resilience for the future. There is a silver lining to what seem like terrible situations! I do not imply that we should seek out stressors, simply that we should reflect on them and use them to broaden our strengths . . . in other words, to build resilience.

Some of the interviews Marcy writes about in this book are with people who fit the definition of frail. Yet you probably can't tell by reading their story, because they have used art, purpose, and other methods to maintain their vitality despite physical challenges. They can be thought of as role models for resilience.

Hugh was in his 70s and working on the biography of a famous violinist when he realized he was taking too many pills, feeling confused, and having difficulty getting in and out of a chair or up and down a few steps – in a word, he was becoming frail. He recognized that he could sink into disability and decided he was not going to do that. He decided he would ride his bike 80 miles on his 80th birthday in 8 hours. At first, this seemed crazy – but he started training. He shed pills and his brain became clearer. His rides grew longer and longer – not without some discomfort! And on his 80th birthday, he accomplished his goal: he hit the 80-mile marker in less than 8 hours.

Frailty is something we are all at risk of developing as we age. But like Hugh, it is *not* a given. Neither is significant loss of our muscles as we grow older. We *can* do something to prevent it. And the best time to start? *Now.*

17 THE WONDERFUL WORLD OF MICROBIOTA AND THE VALUE OF THE MEDITERRANEAN DIET

Elizabeth Eckstrom, MD, MPH, MACP

A common saying we've heard for years is: *"You are what you eat."*

There is more truth in that old adage than most of us realize. Added to that, there is a second part to it that science is recently proving: *"What you eat shapes how you age."*

To see what I mean, let me take you on a virtual tour. It starts in Ostuni, Italy, where I journeyed to learn about how Italy became the healthiest country in the world, with some of the longest-living residents. From there, we will go to a Lilliputian land, as Gulliver did on his travels. We will travel inside the human body to the tiniest world of the microbiota community that lives inside our intestines.

In 2017, researchers from around the world gathered in the Puglia region of southern Italy to attend an international conference where exciting studies on the Mediterranean diet, a nutrition regimen proven to improve longevity, were shared. This pattern of eating, abounding with fruits and vegetables, reduces the chance of developing heart disease, cancer, and other causes of disease and mortality. For many diseases, the Mediterranean diet is better at reducing their risk than any pills doctors can prescribe!

What is it about this diet many Italians enjoy that makes it so protective? How does it work? And why is it important for us to understand?

Because 80% of Americans (and many people in other parts of the world) are *not* eating the foods they need to give them these benefits.

Life depends on consuming food. And do we ever! People ingest an average of 80 tons of food in their lifetimes. (Whoever would have thought?) Childhood obesity predicts early mortality, so a healthy diet needs to start at birth. Beginning a Mediterranean diet early can bestow life-long advantages.

Named for the region where it was identified, the Mediterranean diet consists of simple and often inexpensive foods. Its composition is predominantly vegetarian. Most of the protein in the diet – at least 70% – comes from non-animal sources such as beans, grains, rice, and nuts. It's packed with colorful fresh vegetables and fruits and, researchers note, it seems to be "swimming" in olive oil. Animal fats are discouraged, but eating fish – especially salmon and those rich in omega-3 fatty acids – is of value as the omega-3 fatty acids reduce inflammation, lower blood pressure, and decrease risk factors for disease.

What does that mean for the meat lovers among us? They can take comfort in practicing a common refrain we often hear: moderation in all things. Enjoying chicken breast or lean cuts of beef or lamb a few times a month is perfectly acceptable. But so, too, is being a complete vegetarian. Einstein, Voltaire, Plato, Tolstoy, Da Vinci, and many other famous people were vegetarians – so obviously there is something good about it for our brains!

Patients often wonder: is red wine part of the Mediterranean diet? The answer is a qualified yes. The Mediterranean diet typically allows red wine, also in moderation. Hippocrates, in 480 BC, was correct when he wrote: *Wine is appropriate for the healthy and ailing man.* Wine contains flavonoids and non-flavonoids that are known to be healthy. The polyphenolic component – commonly referred to as dietary antioxidants – found in red wine is associated with decreased cardiovascular disease, diabetes, Alzheimer Disease, and cancer. For most healthy people, one drink per day for women and two for men – *no more* – may allow healthful benefits.

The Mediterranean diet isn't only about the specific foods you ingest. Researchers now understand that your whole eating pattern also appears to contribute to longevity. In countries where the Mediterranean diet is followed, where people live the longest, it is a way of life, one that includes exercise – walking every day – and taking a rest in the afternoon after an enjoyable family meal.

Studies continue to document positive protections this diet offers. As well as contributing to longer lifespans, and reducing the risk of heart disease, cancer, and dementia as we age, newer research shows adhering to the Mediterranean diet can be highly beneficial in managing **diabetes**. For those needing to lose weight for their health, consuming cruciferous vegetables, such as broccoli, cauliflower, and Brussels sprouts, as well as greens and berries, is the most beneficial method for weight loss – more effective than low-fat or low-carbohydrate diets. Equally compelling, newly diagnosed diabetics who followed the Mediterranean diet reduced their risk of needing hypoglycemic medication.

Still another exceptional outcome is the diet's effect on **pain** and **frailty**, both of which can negatively impact our quality of life. Committed adherence to the Mediterranean diet reduces the pain of osteoarthritis – a type of arthritis that occurs when protective tissue at the ends of our bones wears down, and a condition many people develop as they grow older. Frailty, also, can be a serious problem in aging (see Chapter 16). Following the Mediterranean diet has been shown to reduce the risk of developing frailty by as much as 70%!

You may wonder, just what is it that makes the Mediterranean diet so healthful and protective? Like a fascinating twist in a mystery story, its secret is its "toxicity" – a surprising fact which gives it its superpower.

Organisms that exist in harsh environments develop complex mechanisms to cope with environmental stressors. This concept is called *hormesis*. The Mediterranean diet is linked to hormesis because vegetables have some toxic characteristics. If eaten regularly, the low-dose "toxicity" increases your body's resilience and lends protection against chronic diseases.

Where does all this happen in your body? Now it's time to explore that fascinating terrain inside your intestines.

While you are scarcely aware of it, within your intestines there is an ongoing, miniature, teeming world of life. Millions of intestinal microbiota (bacteria) reside there and play essential roles. Beyond helping to digest your food, your intestinal microbiota regulate your immune system and protect against invading bacteria that can cause disease. Fascinating studies show autoimmune diseases, thought to be passed in families, may be the result of a shared microbiome.

Food consumption is the most important contributor to changes in gut microbiota. The Mediterranean diet promotes a highly diverse and advantageous microbiota community, which significantly impacts health in constructive ways. Those older Italians? Studies of the intestinal microbiome of "super centenarians" – people between 105 and 110 years of age – reveal their similarity to those of younger people, rather than those of old people.

The intestinal microbiota has been found to be highly adaptable. If you change your diet, your intestinal world will rapidly change – in a matter of days to weeks! That is good news. It means if you have not been following the Mediterranean diet, start now. Your microbiome could begin protecting you from risk of disease within just 2–3 weeks.

With such obvious advantages, why don't more people eat the Mediterranean diet? Part of the reason, quite simply, is that many still believe it doesn't taste as good. In the United States, it can sometimes be hard to find fresh vegetables and fruits to put on your table, or even in the school lunchroom – especially for people on a limited budget. It requires choosing cheaper vegetables that are less familiar (like bok choy) or on sale, buying whole grains, lentils, and beans in bulk, and knowing how to create fresh crisp salads and cook these items into savory stews and soups.

Recognizing these obstacles, this is what I offer my patients: if at all possible, grow a vegetable garden! Taste and see! Plant easy to grow foods, so you can eat fresh tomatoes, herbs, peppers, arugula, and other delicious staples. Go to your local market and hunt out vegetables and fruit. The diet is not hard to follow, and it's not too complicated to cook. There are many wonderful recipes and it is fun to make up your own. At the back of this book (in the Appendix) are some examples I have created that our family loves and that are easy to make.

Remember, try to get *five colors a day*. Fruits and vegetables make up a vibrant, multihued kaleidoscope! Think spinach, peaches, blueberries, tomatoes, kale, oranges, squash, green beans, sugar snap peas in the shell, broccoli, cauliflower, Brussels sprouts, raspberries. And best of all? Your microbiota will be lively and pleased. They will work to help you and your family achieve longer life, and to perform the roles they were made for: keepers of our health.

18 WHAT HAPPENS TO THE IMMUNE SYSTEM AS WE AGE?

Elizabeth Eckstrom, MD, MPH, MACP

Our immune system is our own personal bodyguard. It is what defends us against foreign invaders seeking to attack our bodies and inflict disease. And it is a system unlike any other: it both destroys and neutralizes infected and malignant cells and removes their debris.

In short, our immune system is our greatest ally when it comes to protecting us from harm. This stealth fighter works around the clock to distinguish our tissue from unfamiliar tissue, our self from non-self. It is composed of myriad units all performing together in one complex, impressive line of defense – from external barriers, like our skin and mucous membranes, to sentries deep within our bodies, such as white blood cells, spleen, lymph nodes, stem cells, and antibodies.

The external, or physical, barriers form our first shields. Our skin itself is a great first fortification – intact skin prevents all sorts of bacteria, viruses, and other harmful agents from getting into our bodies. When we have a cold virus, we often sneeze; if we cut our finger, it may get inflamed. All of these first security systems comprise our *innate immune system*.

Sometimes, however, these defenders aren't enough. An organism such as a bacteria or virus enters our body. We then develop a fever, signaling our immune system is ramping up. What is happening is that our *active immune system* is coming into play. The amazing thing about these reinforcements? They have a memory. They can recall viruses that have invaded before, and can quickly engage and subdue them if they show up again.

That is the basis of one of the greatest feats of modern medicine: the development of vaccines. A vaccine works by "training" our immune system to recognize hostile viruses and bacteria. Vaccines introduce, in a safe manner, small amounts of a pathogen, or antigen, to trigger our body's own immune response, and create antibodies, so it will know how to identify a barrage of antigens at a later time. If the invaders come, our immune system will be called to active duty, and immediately attack and neutralize them before the pathogen can spread and cause illness.

Taken all together, our immune system is designed to fight off infections, heal our wounds, and protect us from malignancy and autoimmune disease. We all know it is not always successful. Things that can hurt us do slip by this amazing fortress, and sometimes even encourage it to respond in ways unintended and damaging to us. Yet the immune system remains our body's chief advocate.

Like all the other systems of our body, this system changes progressively through our lives. Unfortunately, its performance and skills of detection wane as we grow older. This makes us more vulnerable to infections. Some of these effects are inevitable. Others are not. There are things we can do to protect our immune system and mitigate some of the normal forces of aging. In other words, we can help "guard our guardian," which becomes especially important when we reach 70 and older.

In order to understand this terrific system, this chapter has some pretty technical words. Hang in there. I will explain them and, by increasing your understanding, you will learn what you can do to lessen aging changes.

What are these cells primed to fight off invading viruses and infections?

The heroes are our *T cells* and *B cells*. Both are types of white blood cells, called lymphocytes. T cells are produced in the bone marrow and mature in the thymus gland. B cells mature in the bone marrow and are activated in the lymph nodes and spleen. They respond when infected cells send out "distress signals," and are trained and equipped to recognize invaders and muster an offensive.

B cells pump out antibodies that can bind to free viruses and attack them. **T cells** are the generals. They can directly kill cells infected by viruses (and cancer!) and they release proteins called *cytokines* that also help kill virus-infected cells.

Most of the time, B cells and T cells work well and in our favor. There are occasions, though, when things go awry. One such problem is "*autoimmune* disease." These are illnesses that occur when the body mistakenly identifies its own tissues as "foreign" – unable to differentiate "self" from "non-self" – and administers an immune response of "seek and destroy" against them. Examples are multiple sclerosis and rheumatoid arthritis.

Another complication – one we hear about in some patients with COVID-19 – is an overzealous immune system that has "gone rogue." These *cytokine storms*, while not fully understood, create havoc in the immune response. Whether due to genetic factors or unchecked viral infections, they begin striking everything in sight. They begin to raid even healthy cells, to our peril.

We depend on our cytokines to protect us, but in these cases, when the danger is passed they still don't quit attacking. It's an immune system malfunction, and it can be deadly. Thankfully, it is a rare response. Our immune system's main function is to keep us alive.

What exactly happens to our immune system as we age? Quite simply, some of our stalwart guards become less effective.

Scientists describe what occurs as "immunosenescence." It results from decreasing amounts *of hematopoietic stem cells.* These are immature cells that can develop into all types of blood cells, such as white blood cells, red blood cells, and platelets, and are produced in the bone marrow. Why do these cells decrease as we grow older? The reduction is thought to be due to something that happens to our *telomeres.*

Telomeres are protective coverings at the end of each strand of DNA. They shield our chromosomes. I love this definition of them: "Telomeres are like the plastic tips at the end of shoelaces. Without the coating, shoelaces become frayed until they can no longer do their job, just as without telomeres, DNA strands become damaged and our cells can't do their job."

Along with a drop in hematopoietic stem cells, our T and B cells also fall off in number as we age. This results in decreased antibody and immune responses if a new antigen is introduced. But realize, this is all part of normal aging!

Yet, for that reason, anyone over 70 has increased vulnerability to influenza and other infections. Our guards are declining in number. That is why it is critically important that older people get flu shots, COVID shots, pneumonia shots, shingles shots, and keep up with tetanus shots.

Sadly, these normal aging changes can also mean older people have less response to vaccines. So don't wait: it is essential to get pneumonia, shingles, and other important vaccines before you are too old. Get them when they are recommended. Why? In this way, you build up good antibody responses for the future when you may need them the most. Flu shots are required every year because the influenza virus has the ability to evolve, and each year the immunization is modified to respond to the evolution of the virus – and, yes, there is a "high-dose" flu shot that people over 65 should receive. COVID vaccines will likely become a shot that we need to receive on a regular basis, and especially as we age.

There are other reasons older people have a decline in their immune system. Some of these can be reversed. Malnutrition is terrible for our immune systems. Concentrating on maintaining a healthy diet is critical to the vigor of our immune system. Cancer and cancer drugs, drugs that suppress the immune system (such as prednisone and drugs for rheumatoid arthritis), removal of your spleen, HIV, diabetes, and liver and kidney disease all impair immune function, so I encourage you to manage these problems as well as possible.

Another important item to be aware of is that older adults often have *atypical symptoms of infection*. Because of immunosenescence, many older adults don't get a fever when they develop an infection. They can have pneumonia, a gall bladder infection, a urinary tract infection, or other serious medical problems, and still not have an elevated temperature. This happens because many older people have lost the ability to mount an *inflammatory cytokine response* – which is responsible for fever and other things that let you know you are sick! So if an older person has general malaise (just feeling lackluster, new weakness, loss of appetite, discomfort), stops doing their usual activities fairly suddenly, and has new or increased confusion, *be aware* it is possible they have pneumonia, urinary tract infection, or some other infection causing their symptoms!

What are the things we can do to keep our immune systems healthy for as long as we can? Seven actions in particular can help strengthen our bodyguards as they put on a united front to protect us from illness.

1 Maintain proper nutrition throughout your life. Following the Mediterranean diet has been shown to activate the immune response (see Chapter 17).

2 Exercise. You have heard this prescription from me in nearly every chapter I write. Exercise supports a heathy brain and body, and its benefits can't be overstated.

3 Keep up-to-date on your vaccinations. Those recommended for adults 65 and older include:
   • Influenza (annually)
   • Tdap (booster every ten years)
   • Shingles (the Shingrix vaccine, a series of two vaccines for those over 50)
   • Pneumococcal polysaccharide (PPSV23) at 65
   • COVID frequency still being determined

4. Practice good hand hygiene. This is infection prevention at its most basic and best. Studies show good hand-washing reduces the number of people who get sick with diarrhea by 23–40%. Additionally, it reduces diarrheal illness in people with weakened immune systems by 58%. Even more, it has been shown to reduce respiratory illnesses, such as colds, in the general population by 16–21%!

5 Get a good night's sleep. Research shows our T cells go down in number if we are sleep deprived. Lack of sleep can influence whether we come down with a cold or flu, and also how we fight illnesses.

6   Stress is not always a bad thing. But if it lasts too long, it can
     weaken our immune response. Scientists note that when we
     are under constant stress, our T and B cells have more
     difficulty responding to unwelcome invaders. Whenever
     possible, try to lower stress levels.
7   Practice optimism. Our attitude not only can help us see
     things in more positive lights, it also is known to strengthen
     our cell-mediated immunity. Studies conducted by University
     of Kentucky psychology professor Suzanne Segerstrom have
     found that older people who focused on positive information
     were more likely to have stronger immune systems.

The next time you feel that sniffle coming on, think for a moment
of the amazing things your body is doing for you without your
even knowing. Your unsung immune system is working non-stop
to give you a prize beyond measure: protecting your life.

19 THE PROBLEM OF PAIN IN OLDER ADULTS

And What You Can Do about It

Elizabeth Eckstrom, MD, MPH, MACP

You don't have to be very old to start having symptoms of stiffness in the morning, joint aches after activity, and extended pain after even a minor injury. Approximately half of people over 65 have pain that limits their daily function, and pain may worsen homeostenosis (the gradual decline in physiologic reserve with aging that can predispose to frailty). Pain can lead to problems with sleep, mobility, falls, depression, appetite, social isolation, and memory.

There are many reasons older adults have pain. Major culprits are arthritis, neuropathy (nerve pain), headaches, poor teeth (really!), injuries and fractures, back problems – and the list goes on. Is pain a normal part of aging, and just something we have to get used to as we age? Is it better just to "tolerate" pain? Is it better to take pain medication? Will pain just continue to get worse as we get older?

With careful attention, the answer to all of these can be "no."

While there are normal changes with aging that make us more vulnerable to pain, if we are proactive about ways to manage and reduce pain – and don't get unlucky with some terrible accident or painful disease (I will talk about these too) – we can live into very old age reasonably pain free.

Let's discuss each of these questions in more detail.

1   **Is pain a normal part of aging?**
        No, but many problems that are common with aging cause pain. If you start young to prevent aging-related

illnesses, however, you will have a much better chance of
remaining pain free as you age. Here are a few examples of
medical problems that cause pain – and ways to prevent
them.

a   **Arthritis** This widespread problem with aging is best
    prevented by a balanced exercise program that includes
    strength and flexibility training. Arthritis is largely
    a result of too much force being applied repeatedly to our
    joints for years, leading to joint enlargement, decreased
    range of motion, and joint deformity. Strong muscles
    "unweight" the joints, meaning the muscles do more of
    the work so the joints don't have to bear so much applied
    force. Having strong muscles will help reduce the chance
    that your joints will develop arthritis! The catch is that
    strengthening needs to happen to ALL the muscles. For
    example, if all you do is run, you will strengthen your
    hamstrings but not your quadriceps, and your knees will
    get arthritis due to the imbalanced muscles. Biking and tai
    chi both strengthen the quads, making running / biking /
    tai chi a great combination to reduce the risk of knee
    arthritis.

       When I was in my 30s, I loved to run, but started
    having knee pain after running. I didn't want to develop
    arthritis, and began going to the gym to do leg-
    strengthening exercises. I also started biking more and
    doing tai chi. Twenty-five years later, I can still run, bike,
    and do tai chi completely pain free – all because I adopted
    a well-balanced exercise routine as a young adult.

b   **Nerve Pain, or Neuropathy** This is a common cause of
    pain in older adults and is often due to diabetes. Spinal
    stenosis (narrowing of the spinal canal due to arthritic
    changes in the spine) can also cause nerve pain in the legs.
    Once neuropathy develops, it is very hard to reverse. It is
    much better, therefore, to prevent it in the first place!
    Maintaining a healthy weight, following the
    Mediterranean diet, and exercising regularly are the best
    approaches to preventing diabetes – especially if you have

it in your family. It is never too early to start with these healthy practices. More and more children are developing diabetes and they may suffer a lot of neuropathic pain as they age.

c **Chronic Low Back Pain** This is a terrible problem that causes lost days of work (sometimes forcing early retirement), decreased mobility, depression, and even opioid addiction. Back pain can be due to arthritis, spinal canal narrowing (as noted above), muscle tightness, spinal compression fractures, overuse from too much lifting, and many other reasons. Again, the best treatment is prevention. This requires really good core strengthening (think back to the notion that strong muscles help "unweight" the joints). Yoga, tai chi, Pilates, and other core-strengthening regimens are key to preventing back problems as we age. Many people who have back problems will be good about their exercises for a few weeks or months, but when the pain improves, they slack off on the exercises. That is a bad idea! The pain will just return worse than ever. See a physical therapist who specializes in back pain and get a good routine, and then do it every day for the rest of your life.

I have patients in their 80s and 90s who have spine studies such as X-rays or MRIs showing terrible arthritis and other problems, but they have absolutely no pain and can do whatever they want to do. Why is that? They are doing a good back program that prevents back pain. It is totally worth it.

2 **Is it better just to "tolerate" pain? Is it better to take pain medication?**

My answer to both of these is *no*! People who leave their pain untreated often limit their mobility, social interaction, and community engagement because their pain is too severe. This leads to frailty, cognitive decline, falls, and even death. On the other hand, pain medications such as opioids often cause sedation, falls, memory loss, and other dangerous side effects (more about this below). For all these reasons,

I recommend a comprehensive pain reduction strategy, led by your primary care provider, that may include some or all of these:

a   **Movement** This therapy should by now be obvious. Our bodies were built to move 12 miles per day. (I confess – I rarely move that much! Though I certainly try.) If we don't move enough, our muscles stiffen up, our joints lose their mobility, and we have pain. That's why so many older people wake with pain in the morning but feel better after being up for an hour or so. Being still all night triggers pain, which improves as soon as we are up and moving. I am not saying you should get up at night and exercise. However, I am saying it *is* perfectly normal to expect some pain on first awakening – get moving right away to help it go away.

Each week should include at least 30 minutes of aerobic exercise daily, 3 days of strength training for 30 minutes (yoga, Pilates, weights), and 3 days of flexibility training for 30 minutes (tai chi).

b   **Heat** Heat is an amazing pain reliever for older people because it helps reduce the stiffness, decreased mobility, and muscle and joint inflammation related to aging. It feels good while you have the heating pad on a sore back or knee, but it is also helping to *take away* inflammation! If you apply heat regularly at least 4 times daily to sore muscles or joints, over time it can help to reduce pain from arthritis and other common conditions of aging.

c   **Massage, Meditation, and Acupuncture** For many people, these interventions can lead to significant pain reduction, and I strongly encourage utilizing these strategies if they are available to you.

d   **Topical Medications** I strongly encourage people to try topical treatments to see if these will be helpful. Many people get some relief from these medications. Aspercreme® and Icy Hot® and similar over-the-counter topical medications help some people. My favorites, though, are Lidocaine® cream or patches, and diclofenac

(Voltaren® in the US, Voltarol® in the UK) 1% gel.
Lidocaine® is similar to the medication your dentist uses
to numb your teeth for dental work, and is very effective
for nerve pain. Both the cream and the patch are available
without prescription, and can be left on for 12 hours at
a time.

Diclofenac gel is a topical treatment that many of
my patients call "magic goo." It is also over-the-counter,
and widely available. It is an anti-inflammatory medication that gets into joint spaces and doesn't become
absorbed into the blood stream. It acts like ibuprofen or
Aleve® but without the side effects! Many of the smaller
joints that cause pain (in our fingers, elbows, and feet)
don't have great blood supply, so pills don't really get to
those joints very well. Diclofenac gel does. The important
thing is to use it four times daily for several weeks for it to
be really effective, and keep using it to prevent recur-
rence of pain. You must rub it on and then not wash the
area or cover it with clothes for 10 minutes to allow it to
soak in. Diclofenac gel is very safe because it is not
absorbed systemically. This means it is all right to use
even if you are on a blood thinner for atrial fibrillation or
have other reasons not to take oral anti-inflammatory
medications.

e **Safer Oral Pain Medications** Acetaminophen
(paracetamol) is extremely safe for older adults. Many
people have heard it can cause kidney and liver problems.
But if you are not in full kidney failure and don't drink
alcohol excessively, you will likely be able to take
acetaminophen 1000 mg up to three times daily
completely safely for years. While it doesn't help everyone,
it is definitely worth a try of taking it regularly, 1000 mg 3
times daily for a month, to see if it does lead to benefits. If
so, it is much safer than any other pain pills.

f **Oral Medication with Questionable Safety for
Older Adults** Ibuprofen, naproxen, and other anti-
inflammatory drugs MIGHT be safe for some older adults

for a short time. You cannot use them *at all* if you have kidney problems, difficult-to-control high blood pressure, difficult-to-control congestive heart failure, a history of a gastrointestinal bleed, or if you take blood thinners for atrial fibrillation or other reasons. If you don't have any of these contraindications, it may be safe to take these medications for a short time (2–3 weeks) for hip bursitis, a flare of gout, or other acute problems. If your doctor allows you to take one of these medications, be sure they keep track of your blood pressure, leg swelling (limiting salt can eliminate this), and kidney function while you are on them.

Of note: though these medications are risky in older people, research shows that they are much safer than opioid medications such as oxycodone, so they are worth considering if they are possible for you.

9 **Oral Medications with Questionable Safety, but that Might Be Useful in Certain Situations**
Gabapentin is an anti-seizure medication that has good effectiveness for diabetic neuropathy and other nerve pain. It can cause sedation, confusion, and other side effects in older adults, but if used cautiously at low doses (generally 300–600 mg per day maximum), it could relieve pain without significant side effects. It should never be used with opioids. Duloxetine, a good antidepressant, is also fairly safe for older adults and has some pain relief properties. I like to use this for patients with pain and depression.

Oral Medications that I Recommend Avoiding Completely If Possible. Opioid medications such as hydro-codone, oxycodone, and morphine are *very risky* in older adults. They cause confusion, falls, fracture, kidney failure, hospitalization, and even death. In addition, they don't actually help treat pain very much! Many studies of common pain conditions like back pain and arthritis show that opioids are actually no better for pain management than a placebo (fake drug) or non-drug treatments. I completely agree with using opioid medications for cancer pain and other pain at the end of life, but if you have chronic back pain, arthritis pain, irritable bowel syndrome, or other non-cancer types of pain, these drugs will *not help your pain* and will only cause *dangerous side effects.*

3   **Will pain continue to get worse as we age?**

Not necessarily. As I mentioned, people with severe arthritis can live pain free if they are "doing everything right." It is probably not possible to be pain free all day, every day, but with good pain relief strategies, practiced daily, it is possible to do everything you want to do. And *that* is the important consideration: it may not be possible to relieve all your *pain* 100%, but the goal should be to retain 100% of your *function.*

I hope many younger people are reading this while you can still do things to prevent pain when you're older! But even if you are already 90 and suffering from substantial pain, please be hopeful! Working with your primary care provider, physical therapist, exercise trainer, masseuse, acupuncturist, and other team members could dramatically reduce your pain and improve your function.

One of my 80-something patients who had been in a wheelchair for 15 years due to pain from arthritis was motivated to walk again. She started physical therapy, chair tai chi (and later standing tai chi), diclofenac gel and heat four times daily, and weekly massage therapy. After a year, she could walk a quarter of a mile, and her pain was reduced on a 'scale of 1 to 10' from 8 to 3.

She had the most beautiful smile when I watched her walk in my office!

20 DON'T GIVE IN AND LIVE WITH PAIN

First, Give Physical Therapy a Try

Darla Philips, PT, DPT, ATC, OCS

There are many fairly obvious, objective benefits to attending physical therapy: increased strength, improved flexibility, and better joint mobility – all of which can lead to decreased pain and increased function. But one of the less obvious advantages frequently can be seen even before a patient's hard work translates into those main physical changes.

That benefit is hope.

People often come into their evaluation discouraged by a poor prognosis from a physician or imaging that reveals more wear and tear on their bodies than they feel they can overcome. Even more, there is a tendency to discount the likelihood that progress can be made in older patients. But that is generally not the case!

The good news is: many people can make significant gains even when their radiographs show joints that are bone on bone or lumbar discs that are no longer as hydrated as they once were. Physical therapy can provide a plan to give patients control over an injury or pathology that previously felt unmanageable. This is especially true among older adults.

Giving a patient a strategy for pain management as well as home exercises to work on impairments (strength, flexibility, or mobility) allows them to transition from feeling like a victim, betrayed by their body, to a person empowered to halt these unwanted changes.

While I acknowledge that one must be realistic about the amount of change you can induce if there are deficits present (even with depressing imaging), gains can be made.

Here's why. X-rays or MRIs showing degenerative changes don't account for pain that is caused by *flexibility and strength deficits or poor movement patterns*. These are things which can be addressed and corrected with physical therapy! While it is true that strength gains happen more slowly in people who are not young and spry, they can still be made if consistent exercises are performed. Even more, correcting a patient's biomechanics can take the burden off arthritic joints and facilitate pain-free movement.

An example of a person who has overcome the odds is an 86-year-old patient of mine. When she first began physical therapy, she was experiencing lower back pain at a level of 8 out of 10 while using a walker. Her physician had told her she would never walk again without pain. He said her only options were to continue to use a walker, transition to a wheelchair, or undergo a surgery he was not certain she would survive.

Her imaging gave validation to her doctor's supposition. X-rays showed significant osteoarthritis and an anterior shift in her lumbar spine which, in combination with the patient's level of pain and her age, drove the physician's grim prognosis.

But the imaging did not reveal everything. What it could not show was the patient's significant deficits of flexibility in her anterior hip musculature and her core, and lower-extremity weakness, all of which were creating shearing forces on her lumbar spine, and leading to poor static posture and an inability to bend or lift properly.

So there was indeed something that could be done to relieve her pain, without forcing her to live with discomfort or be wheelchair-bound for the rest of her life. She chose to give physical therapy a try. Together, we worked out a combination of manual therapy techniques, neuromuscular re-education, therapeutic exercises, and patient education.

Today this patient can comfortably walk in her community with only a hiking pole to assist with balance!

While physical therapy is not a magic cure for all that ails us, it can facilitate meaningful gains by addressing musculoskeletal impairments. These changes, in combination with guidance to correct biomechanical faults, can lead to decreased pain during work and household tasks. Even more, it can allow for a safe return to many desired hobbies and exercise programs, and a subsequent improvement in quality of life.

PART III
Caring For Yourself and Your Family

Practical Planning

Tomorrow belongs to the people who prepare for it today.

African proverb

21 WHO NEEDS AN ESTATE PLAN? EVERYONE

Wendy K. Goidel, Esq.

(Author's note: The following three chapters are applicable to the legal and financial systems in the United States. Notwithstanding this disclaimer, many of the concepts and considerations discussed are similar throughout the world. Indeed, the goals of estate, long-term care, financial, and retirement planning are agnostic. While some of the names of the estate planning documents referred to in this chapter may differ among countries, the purpose for each is similar. Other factors such as a jurisdiction's estate, gift, and income tax rules and rates can affect or dictate estate planning options. It should also be noted that qualification for government funding of all or a portion of long-term care costs is not only country-specific, but typically differs by locality. But since most programs are means-tested, proactive asset protection planning may be required. No matter the type of planning required or desired, there is no substitute to consulting with qualified estate planning and financial advisors in your locale about your specific situation, needs, and goals.)

Confusion about the term "estate planning" may be due to its first word: *estate*. An estate conjures up images of large country manors, villas with manicured gardens and vineyards, palatial homes, and, of course, lots of money. While most of us work hard to cover our monthly expenses and save what is left for retirement, we will never own this type of property. Thus, we mistakenly conclude that we do not need to engage in estate planning. However, nothing could be further from the truth.

In fact, every adult needs an estate plan, regardless of age, race, religion, culture, or wealth. Simply put, an estate plan is a set of legal written instructions stating how you want to be cared for, how your assets should be spent if you become incapacitated, and how and to whom your assets should be distributed after you die. Assets include your home, bank accounts, retirement accounts, life insurance policies, and personal property. A properly designed estate plan covers the following phases of your life:

- When you are alive and well, your estate plan will allow you to have full access to and stay in total control of your assets. Studies show that loss of financial autonomy corresponds to a decline in physical, emotional, and mental health. Thus, your plan should allow you to remain in control of your assets for as long as possible, as that is critical to maintaining good health.

- If you become mentally incapacitated, either temporarily or permanently, your estate plan will provide instructions to the agents you name, who will make your legal, financial, and medical decisions. Your plan will guide them as to how and where you want to be cared for and how your assets should be spent and protected.

- When you die, your estate plan will leave your assets to your loved ones or other beneficiaries with clear instructions as to how and when they will receive distributions. Depending upon the type of planning, the instructions can remain private and eliminate the expense and delay of court involvement.

Discussions about incapacity and death are neither comfortable nor easy. Obviously, nobody knows if or when they may become incapacitated. However, everyone knows that death is certain. If only we had that crystal ball to advise when these events will happen.

What we do have, however, is a choice of when and how to plan. We can choose to plan proactively or reactively. The optimal time to start planning is when you are relatively young and healthy. This is called proactive estate planning. At this stage of your life, you can make your own decisions, create your own instructions, remain in complete control, and have full access to your assets. You can also protect all or a portion of your assets in the event of incapacity. This can be accomplished without pressure, on your schedule and terms, and without the anxiety and worry caused by illness or incapacity. If you later become ill or incapacitated, your estate plan will guide your family as to how to care for you and manage your property. And when you die, your family will be grateful that you provided a roadmap for the administration of your estate.

Studies show a direct correlation between the quality of life of those who are suffering from illness or incapacity and their level of planning. Creating a clear and comprehensive plan is truly a gift to your loved ones.

What if you do not have an estate plan and you suffer a significant health crisis? You will fall into the category of reactive estate planning. In this case, you may not be the one making the decisions and providing the instructions. This is typically because you have a condition that affects your cognitive ability. In this situation, your loved ones or designated agents are scrambling to meet with an estate planning or elder-law attorney to create some semblance of a plan. *You may not even be in the conference room* during the planning. Based upon the severity of your illness or condition, you are probably at home receiving care, in a hospital or rehabilitation facility, or residing in a skilled-nursing home. At this point, it is probably impossible to protect most or all of your assets. And it is also easy for your loved ones to become frustrated about your failure to plan. They are pressured to make the right decisions for you, and stressed about managing your difficult health issues and care needs.

This is not the legacy anyone should leave to family or friends.

Admittedly, nobody rushes out to meet for coffee with friends or relatives to discuss death and disability. It is understandable to deflect and discuss just about any other topic or issue. However, the dialogues between you, your loved ones, and an estate planning attorney can help you address and plan for unforeseen events and avoid unintended negative consequences. Failing to properly plan can result in expensive errors and preventable problems. Making the difficult decisions and signing the necessary legal documents constitutes planning by design rather than default.

There are several issues to consider before commencing the estate planning process. Because an estate plan is comprised of documents containing personal and sensitive information, it should not be thought of as a product or commodity. Even though you can read much about estate planning – true and false – on the Internet, legal documents should not be purchased in a box or online or considered as a "do-it-yourself" project. Estate planning is too important for that. The documents that most people create themselves by answering a series of online questions are typically generic, overly broad, or inadequate to meet their needs and objectives. With so many complex laws and considerations, there is no substitute for having your estate plan designed and drafted by a competent, experienced estate planning and/or elder-law attorney.

If you do not have an estate planning attorney, ask for referrals from your friends, relatives, financial advisor, or accountant. Schedule an initial consultation to assess the attorney's know-ledge, competency, compassion, and empathy. Once you feel comfortable and are ready to proceed, there are several types of conversations you should expect to have with your attorney.

First, before any documents are discussed, there should be a conversation about your goals, needs, values, aspirations, and objectives. There should be discussion and analysis of your health, income, assets, insurance, and – here's the most personal part – family dynamics. Without full disclosure and discussion, your estate plan may not truly work for you or your family. That is why you must be willing to discuss difficult issues and topics, all of which your attorney is required to hold in the strictest of confidence.

This conversation should not be one-sided. After you disclose information about you, your family, and your finances, your attorney should provide you with relevant estate planning information and present different legal strategies and solutions to satisfy *your* specific needs and goals. The information presented should be completely understandable. Never settle for or tolerate an attorney who speaks in legalese. If you do not understand something, ask for clarification. You should leave the initial meeting feeling educated, empowered, and equipped to make the right estate planning decisions for yourself and your family.

Second, your attorney should introduce you to the following principal estate planning documents: (1) Last Will and Testament; (2) Living Trust; (3) Power of Attorney; (4) Health Care Proxy; and (5) Living Will. Depending upon the state of your domicile, these documents may be titled differently. Notwithstanding its name, each document must be designed and tailored to meet your specific needs and family situation. Especially when planning proactively, there is no one-size-fits-all approach; rather, there are different options to be discussed and considered. Each document, as will be discussed below, becomes part of a comprehensive estate plan. Considering your financial situation and goals, the documents can be designed to:

- protect assets from future creditors (including long-term care costs)
- provide for the needs of a surviving spouse (especially in a second marriage)
- provide for liquidity at death (without the need to sell a home or other property)
- promote family harmony (if married, usually upon the death of the surviving spouse)
- protect inheritances for minor children (including those with special needs)
- protect inheritances for adult children (from divorce, creditors, and lawsuits)
- leave or promote a legacy (whether it be financial and/or value-based)
- benefit one or more charitable organizations or foundations
- eliminate or reduce income, estate, or inheritance taxes

Let's build a sample estate plan by discussing each document.

1   Last Will and Testament

The centerpiece of a traditional estate plan consists of a *Last Will and Testament ("Will")*. This document outlines how the executor – the person appointed to administer your estate – must distribute assets to your named beneficiaries – individuals and/or charities – after your death. In most states, Wills are also necessary for the nomination of guardians to care for minor children in the unlikely event of both parents' premature passing.

Sometimes younger parents procrastinate or fail to sign their Wills because of a disagreement over the designation of the appropriate guardians. There may be friction about who would be better suited to raise their children, and concern that family members who are not selected will feel hurt or insulted. While it is important to consult with the proposed guardians to assess their willingness and ability to serve, in addition to their values and child-rearing philosophies, there is no obligation to notify other relatives that they are not being named. And rest assured that your Will can be revised if you decide to change the designated guardians.

Many people believe that a Will is sufficient to satisfy or address their estate planning needs. However, if you are older or do not have minor children, a Will strictly operates as a plan for distributing assets after death. A Will does absolutely nothing for you during your lifetime. The document itself can neither provide for the protection or expenditure of your assets while you are alive, nor determine what happens to you or your assets should you become incapacitated.

Wills were sufficient in the days when lifespans were shorter and death preceded the need for long-term care.

Those days are essentially over. With people living far longer than ever before, our added longevity – while a great benefit – often comes with a corresponding rise in prolonged illness and cognitive impairment. This makes a Will, in the absence of other estate planning documents, entirely inadequate in protecting you and your assets.

It is important to understand that the named executor has no authority to follow the instructions in your Will until it has been admitted to probate. Probate is the legal process by which your Will is submitted to court to have it declared valid and have the named executor appointed. The Will must be probated before the executor can collect and distribute assets which were held in your individual name. If your assets were owned jointly or had designated beneficiaries, there is no reason to probate your Will, as they pass to the joint owner or named beneficiary by operation of law.

As part of the probate process, your heirs (your closest relatives pursuant to law) are required to be notified of your death and the existence of your Will. Regardless of whether they are named as beneficiaries, your heirs are required to consent to the Will or appear in court to object to its validity and/or the appointment of the named executor. Probate is relatively simple if your heirs are competent adults who are being treated equally. However, the process can become especially problematic if your heirs are minors, incapacitated, or are being treated differently or even disinherited. All that is required for a contested probate matter is the failure of one heir to provide the required consent.

Depending upon the state in which you reside, the probate process can be either simple or complicated. Unfortunately, though, in all states, the process inherently results in delay, a loss of privacy, and additional expense. This means that your assets cannot be collected and distributed until the court process is concluded.

A Will is essential to ensure that your assets pass to your intended beneficiaries, either outright or in trust. If you die "intestate" – without a Will – the laws of your domicile will determine who your heirs are and dictate who receives your property. This unintended consequence can easily be avoided by proper planning.

The good news is that the pitfalls of probate and intestacy can be avoided through the creation and funding of Living Trusts. These are private documents which, upon your incapacity or death, do not require court intervention or the consent of family members.

2   Living Trusts

Many people understandably believe that trusts are complicated and costly; however, they can be drafted to ensure simplicity and minimize expense. Let's dispel these misconceptions and demystify the concept of trusts.

There are two main types of trusts: Testamentary Trusts and Living Trusts. A *Testamentary Trust* is one that is created in your Will. Before that trust is effective, two things must occur: (1) you need to die; and (2) your Will must be admitted to probate. That trust can be funded for the benefit of your spouse or other heirs after your executor collects your assets and satisfies your debts, claims, expenses, and estate taxes. Obviously, by its very nature, a testamentary trust does absolutely nothing to protect your assets or provide for you or your family during your lifetime.

However, a *Living Trust* is a legal entity that becomes the "owner" of your assets during your lifetime. It is essentially a contract between three parties: (a) the *creator* of the trust (often referred to as either the trustmaker, trustor, grantor, or settlor); (b) the *trustee* (an individual such as a friend, relative, or accountant) or entity (such as a financial institution) named to manage, invest, and distribute the assets; and (c) the *beneficiaries* (the individuals and entities who may receive distributions of income and/ or principal during and after the creator's lifetime). Depending upon the type of trust, you can be the creator, serve as a trustee, and be a lifetime beneficiary. And, significantly, the trust is a private document which remains with the creator; it is neither required to be filed in court nor recorded with any governmental agency during the creator's lifetime or after death.

The need for a trust is determined by each person's goals, objectives, and aspirations, and – here is the significant part – not by net worth. *Contrary to popular belief, trusts are not relegated to the wealthy; they can be created for and benefit individuals of all income brackets.* They can be drafted to accomplish one, more, or all of the goals and protections discussed above.

There are two main types of Living Trusts – **Revocable** and **Irrevocable**.

A Revocable Living Trust – often referred to as a "Will substi-tute" – takes effect immediately after you sign it. Unlike a traditional Will, a Revocable Living Trust can include detailed instructions for the management, investment, and distribution of your assets during your lifetime and after your death. Thus, the Revocable Living Trust covers the following three phases of your life:

i   While you are alive and well, you are typically the trustee and permitted to stay in control of your assets. You also have total access to the assets, with the power to decide how they should be invested, spent, and distributed. There are no restrictions on your ability to substitute and exchange assets. And, importantly, you can amend or revoke the trust should your needs or circumstances change.

ii   In the event of temporary or permanent incapacity, the trust provides instructions to be followed by your designated successor trustee. The trust should state how your property should be spent on your care, and whether distributions can be made to benefit your spouse or other dependents. If drafted properly, your successor trustee does not have full or unfettered discretion to invest, spend, or distribute your assets. The instructions you create with your estate planning attorney should provide clear parameters or guidelines, permitting the successor trustee to act in your best interests and satisfy your goals and objectives. These can include the authority to gift assets to beneficiaries or transfer assets to irrevocable trusts for tax or long-term care planning purposes.

iii   Upon your death, the trust provides instructions to the successor trustee for the distribution of your assets to named beneficiaries, either outright or in further trust. This should all be achieved outside of the probate process.

To provide the most value and benefit, the Revocable Living Trust should be more than just a Will substitute. Indeed, it should include a full set of instructions to guide the successor trustee in the event of your incapacity. The definition of "incapacity" – and the nomination of individuals who can make that determination – should be included in the trust document. A medical diagnosis is not necessarily required, and your primary care physician need not be consulted. Rather, the determination can be made by your "disability panel" comprised of individuals you select (typically a spouse and adult children) who would recognize if you began showing signs of cognitive impairment. They may be concerned about your mismanagement of trust property, or undue influence being asserted by others. These individuals can act to remove you as a trustee so that your successor trustee can immediately step in to protect you and the trust assets.

While the Revocable Living Trust provides many benefits, it neither protects your assets from future creditors nor minimizes or eliminates estate taxes. To achieve those goals, you may also consider creating an **Irrevocable Trust**. Once assets are transferred into an Irrevocable Trust, you typically cannot serve as the trustee or be a beneficiary. The assets will be retitled in the name of the trust and will no longer be owned by you. While this can provide considerable income and/or estate tax benefits, it does come with a corresponding loss of access to and control over the assets. These types of trusts are usually created for individuals with high net worth, family businesses, and/or charitable intent.

There is, however, a special type of Irrevocable Trust that proves invaluable for long-term care planning purposes.

A **Medicaid Asset Protection Trust**, if properly designed and funded, can protect your assets in advance of needing long-term care. This is especially beneficial for those who lack sufficient income and assets to pay for their long-term care needs or are unwilling or unable to obtain long-term care insurance.

If you are engaging in proactive estate planning, you have the opportunity to protect assets to become financially eligible for the Medicaid program. Medicaid is a federal and state-administered program which may fund all or a portion of your long-term care expenses, either at home or in a skilled-nursing facility. Each state has its own stringent income and asset thresholds which must be met prior to obtaining eligibility. There are many requirements and different lookback periods which must be satisfied. If assets are transferred to the Medicaid Asset Protection Trust sufficiently in advance of needing care, they should not be counted as resources in determining financial eligibility.

While you are the creator of the Medicaid Asset Protection Trust, you typically cannot serve as a trustee and can never be a principal beneficiary. However, you can designate lifetime beneficiaries (individuals other than your spouse) who can receive discretionary distributions of principal if necessary. If you need the income generated from the trust assets to help you satisfy your living expenses, the trustee can be directed to make mandatory or discretionary distributions of income to you and your spouse. And, if ownership of your home is transferred to the trust, you will certainly reserve the right to lifetime use and occupancy, with the corresponding obligation to cover all expenses attendant to the home's maintenance and upkeep. Significantly, the trust is designed to protect assets so that they do not need to be liquidated and drained to cover the cost of exorbitant care. Instead, the trust protects assets so that they can be passed down to your loved ones.

While trusts are more expensive to create during your lifetime strictly due to legal fees, the costs of administration after your death are significantly reduced due to the avoidance of probate. The quantifiable financial savings, and unquantifiable emotional savings, often tip the scales in favor of trust-based planning.

3　Power of Attorney

Whether or not you decide to create and fund a Living Trust, there are several essential legal documents which must accompany your estate plan. Perhaps the most powerful document is the comprehensive durable general Power of Attorney. In this document, you will designate one or more agents to make legal and financial decisions for you should you become incapacitated or unable to act on your own behalf.

The term "comprehensive" means that you have given your agents broad powers to step into your shoes and perform any and all tasks that you could perform if you had the ability to do so.

While the Power of Attorney can be drafted to provide your agents with limited powers or for a specific purpose – such as to represent you at a real estate closing – it will be inadequate should you later become incapacitated and unable to execute a more comprehensive document.

The term "durable" means that the document will survive and be effective in the event of your incapacity. This is significant, as it does not require a medical diagnosis or determination of your incapacity.

When the Power of Attorney is part of a trust-based estate plan, the document empowers the agents to handle legal and financial matters not covered by the trust. The trustee of the trust is granted the power to make all decisions, and transact any business, regarding the assets transferred to the trust. The Power of Attorney merely enumerates the powers granted to the agents over other assets and issues. There is no ability to include specific instructions to guide the agents. Even if your agents want to carry out your instructions should you become incapacitated, they may not know or understand your intent or wishes. For this reason, a trust becomes more significant and valuable, in that it can be designed to provide specific and detailed instructions for the management, investment, and distribution of trust assets.

From a practical standpoint, it is important that you name agents whom you completely trust and who have the required acumen to handle your legal and financial affairs. The agents may be the same individuals whom you name as the trustees of your Living Trust and executors of your Will. While spouses and adult children are often named, the agents can be trusted friends or professional advisors (e.g., attorneys and accountants). Placed in the wrong hands, the Power of Attorney is tantamount to handing a blank check to your agents. While the agents are fiduciaries and legally required to act in your best interests, the document provides full authority over and access to your funds. From an estate and long-term care planning perspective, it is important that the document provide the agents with the ability to create and fund trusts if that becomes warranted and necessary.

The worst-case scenario will arise if you fail to execute a power of attorney and/or trust and later become incapacitated. Without the requisite legal documents, nobody has the power – not even your spouse – to make your legal and financial decisions. The only option is the commencement of a court proceeding for the appointment of a guardian. An individual or entity will submit a petition outlining your situation and the need for the appointment of a guardian for your personal needs and property management. Attorneys may be appointed to represent you and to investigate the need for the appointment of a guardian. Following a trial or hearing in an open courtroom, the judge may declare you as an incapacitated person and specify the powers granted to the guardian. At this juncture, your privacy and dignity have been significantly diminished.

The nature of the proceeding subjects your legal, financial, and personal concerns to scrutiny. While the proceeding is designed to protect vulnerable individuals, it can become extremely intrusive, expensive, and unpleasant. Court-awarded attorneys' fees and expenses will be satisfied from your assets. In addition, the proceeding requires annual reporting of your personal situation and a financial accounting to the court for oversight and approval. And, depending upon your personal situation and family dynamics, the court may appoint an unrelated third party as the guardian over your personal needs and property management. That person, who had no prior relationship with you, may now have the power to make your medical decisions, choose your residence, and manage your property.

These unfortunate results can entirely be avoided through proper proactive estate planning.

4   Health Care Proxy (a.k.a. Health Care Power of Attorney)

The one power that cannot be granted to an agent in a Power of Attorney is the ability to make healthcare decisions on your behalf. Thus, your estate plan must include a Health Care Proxy or Health Care Power of Attorney, also known as a medical advance directive. This document names individuals whom you trust to make healthcare decisions in the event that you become incapacitated or temporarily unable to communicate your wishes.

Often a spouse or life partner and adult child are named as the primary and alternate healthcare agents. However, the choice of agents is critical, and should not be quickly decided solely based on relationship or birth order. Choose your agents with care and after conversations with potential candidates, as it is important that their viewpoints are *congruent with your own and that they completely understand your wishes.* You will want to name individuals who understand your values and wishes, can advocate for necessary and appropriate treatment and intervention, and will ensure that you receive the care and attention you require and deserve.

In addition to naming agents to make your medical decisions, the Health Care Proxy can also indicate your instructions regarding organ donation upon your death. It can clearly state your desire not to donate organs, or it can be specific as to which organs may be donated and to whom.

A properly designed Health Care Proxy will also adhere to the requirements of the Health Information Portability and Accountability Act (HIPAA), giving your agents the ability to obtain your confidential medical information and records.

Rather than signing a Health Care Proxy in a hospital during the admission process when you are stressed out and completing multiple forms, it is preferable to execute a proper document after careful consideration and drafting by your attorney. Unlike the Health Care Proxy signed in a hospital which is hospital-specific, the document that is prepared by your attorney is portable and will be accepted by all medical providers and hospitals. It can always be replaced by an updated document that appoints different agents.

5   Living Will

The one decision that should not be left to your healthcare agent is the decision whether you live or die. Instead, consider creating a Living Will which provides instructions for medical treatment, intervention, and end-of-life care should you be declared terminal or comatose or are determined to be in a persistent vegetative state with no hope of recovery. If either declaration or determination is made, and should you suffer a heart attack or stroke, the document can clearly state that you do not wish to be resuscitated, intubated, or ventilated. These wishes would be your DNR (Do Not Resuscitate), DNI (Do Not Intubate), and DNV (Do Not Ventilate) orders. They can state that you do not want to receive artificial nutrition, respiration, or hydration. The reality is that the intervention of such measures will not restore cognitive function. While those measures may prolong the duration of your life, they will not maintain or enhance your quality of life.

Notwithstanding those directives, the document can state that you wish to be kept comfortable through the administration of pain-alleviating medication. Of course, these decisions require careful thought and consideration. Some individuals may choose to permit certain interventions, should their medical team determine that there is some hope for recovery. Either way, the document should authorize the hospital to withdraw all means of life support without liability for your eventual passing.

A properly designed Living Will should not leave this end-of-life decision making to your healthcare agents. Putting your instructions in writing allows your family or loved ones to grieve and proceed with their own lives, recognizing and finding solace in the fact that they followed your wishes. Certainly, the peace of mind provided through the creation of appropriate instructions is the final gift you can give to your family.

Advance Care Directives

Finally, you can consider creating an additional individualized advance directive – one that is important but not legally enforceable. If you are concerned about developing Alzheimer or another form of dementia, an advance care directive can be drafted by your attorney to provide detailed instructions for your caregivers.

Depending upon the geographical proximity and emotional closeness of your family members, they may be unfamiliar with your living preferences and daily routine. Thus, creating a blueprint or set of instructions – akin to those you might leave with a grandparent or babysitter charged with watching your children – is instrumental in maximizing your independence and enhancing your quality of life.

Indeed, the document can include preferences for how you like to be dressed and groomed, the identity of people and places you enjoy visiting, and particular hobbies and activities that provide pleasure. The document can be detailed to include the genre of books you prefer reading; the newspapers or magazines to which you subscribe; the sports teams you support; the movies, television shows, and music you appreciate; and the religion you may practice. You can also note the specific foods and beverages you like and dislike.

Many people with dementia or Alzheimer Disease may not remember what they prefer to do or eat until it is provided for them. Creating a detailed set of instructions can help your loved ones to make the right decisions about your daily care. While this type of document is not legally enforceable, and takes time to compose, it is far superior to having no instructions in place. Finally, it will also provide you with peace of mind, knowing that you have taken all possible steps to maximize your quality of life.

In *The Gift of Caring*, Marcy Houle discussed the creation of a *Daily Continuity of Care Checklist* for her mother's caregivers. She also designed a *Caregiver's Guide for a Typical Day* to outline her mother's preferences. While her mother did not suffer from dementia, she did need assistance with her activities of daily living. Undoubtedly, both tools improved her mother's quality of life.

Lastly, the type of instructions you create when you are young and healthy will differ greatly from those you will need when you are older and facing health issues and care needs.

The following are some planning suggestions through the decades.

Twenties through Forties

At minimum, during your *20s through 40s,* you will need a foundational estate plan consisting of a Will, Power of Attorney, Health Care Proxy, and Living Will. Many individuals sign their first estate plan after the birth of their first child. Of course, trust-based planning may also be desired and needed for asset protection and probate avoidance.

Fifties through Sixties

These are the decades when many individuals start to consider asset protection and long-term care planning. They may have been named as executors in their parents' Wills and experienced the pitfalls of probate. They may have also witnessed their parents' spend-down of assets on long-term care. Desiring to avoid similar issues, they may better understand the concept and benefits of trust-based planning. Notwithstanding whether a Will or Living Trust is the centerpiece of the estate plan, all documents should be reviewed and updated based on changes in your health, wealth, family members, obligations, taxes, and the laws.

Seventies through Nineties

In your 70s through 90s, things get more complicated and critical. If you have neither started nor updated your planning, time is now of the essence. Even if you are relatively healthy, having a current estate plan is critical. Nobody can predict the onset of a catastrophic health event. Further, the window of opportunity to execute estate planning documents quickly closes if cognitive impairment begins, and rises to the level of legal incapacity.

At this time in your life, the basic estate planning documents required during earlier decades remain the same, but the conversation changes. Discussions about protecting family members and planning for your care usually are very different. For those who have long-term care insurance and/or sufficient income and assets to fund their care, a Revocable Living Trust typically becomes the central estate planning document. For others, a Medicaid Asset Protection Trust often becomes the centerpiece of a sound estate plan.

A comprehensive estate plan is essential to meet your current and future needs, regardless of your age. Working closely with your attorney and other advisors, you can design documents that address your financial, legal, tax, and care needs. Your plan can afford you the opportunity to live comfortably, ensure financial security for your loved ones after you die, and protect the assets you leave to your loved ones, while promoting your financial and emotional values.

After signing your documents, you can rest assured that you have provided not only for the quality of *your* life, but also for the lives of those you love.

Consider taking the following eight estate planning steps:

1   Outline your estate planning needs, goals, aspirations, and wishes.
2   Consult with an attorney specializing in estate planning or elder law.
3   Choose the right agents, executors, and trustees to carry out your instructions.
4   At a minimum, sign a Last Will and Testament, Power of Attorney, Health Care Proxy, and Living Will.
5   Design a blueprint for your care should you become cognitively impaired.
6   Consider creating a Living Trust for asset protection and probate avoidance.
7   Store your estate planning documents in a secure location and tell your family members and agents where they are located in the event of your incapacity and death.
8   Create lists of your assets, account numbers, passwords, and PIN numbers, and store them with your estate planning documents.

22 FINANCIAL PLANNING THROUGH THE DECADES

Wendy K. Goidel, Esq.

Gone are the days when workers planned for a hard stop at age 65, collected Social Security and a pension, and lived leisurely for another 5 to 15 years. Gone, too, are those "golden" years when many people did not worry about outliving funds or hemorrhaging savings to pay for expensive and protracted long-term care. Life was simpler then.

Enter the twenty-first century.

Today, trying to achieve a work–life balance while ensuring financial stability has become much more difficult. With increasing longevity, coupled with concerns about the stability of Social Security and the scarcity of pensions, many in the workforce face pressures to remain employed well past the traditional retirement age or their original expectations.

Studies indicate that most people approaching retirement are neither financially nor emotionally prepared to stop working. According to the Brookings Institute Retirement Security Project, nearly half of all workers do not have access to employer-sponsored or traditional pensions. Many small business owners and entrepreneurs, particularly, face the need to increase savings, invest wisely, and create their own pensions. The failure to recognize and plan for a potential gap between savings and expected longevity creates additional stress.

Added to that, over the past 50 years, the concept of financial planning for retirement has undergone an extreme metamorphosis. And it hasn't been a positive change.

In the 1950s through the early 1970s, most Americans were typically tethered to one employer – who was loyal to them – for their entire careers. With that loyalty often came a pension which, when coupled with Social Security, made it unnecessary for an employee to accumulate assets in any substantial way.

As a result of myriad economic challenges in the 1970s, the connection between employer and employee became fractured, and along with it the pension component of a retirement plan. Even where an employer still maintained a pension plan, its ultimate benefits might have been significantly reduced.

Currently, it is almost impossible to rely solely on the government or an employer to fund your retirement lifestyle. Instead, you need to create your own sound financial plan. It is important to consider and plan for your individual goals and priorities, your work–life balance, and what opportunities are available to supplement your earnings during your working years to fund a secure retirement.

Successful retirement, more than ever, requires proper planning through the decades, starting in your 20s and continuing through your 70s.

Financial Planning in your Twenties

The key to saving enough for retirement is to invest as much as possible, as early as possible.

The bottom line is this: you must create an investment strategy where you literally do not run out of money before you die.

A retirement plan's best friend is the concept of compounding. In order to understand this concept, you must first learn *the Theory of 72*.

The Theory of 72, while sounding complicated, is actually relatively straightforward. More than anything, it is simple math: if you divide 72 by an assumed rate of return, you will learn how long it takes for an investment to double.

For example, if you purchase a mutual fund for $10,000 touting an annual 6% rate of return, it will take 12 years for that investment to turn into $20,000 (72/6 = 12). At a heady 8% return, doubling will occur in 9 years, while at a rather paltry 4% return, it will take 18 years for the investment to double.

Affecting any rate of return are investment fees and inflation. Assuming a 1% investment fee and a 3% rate of inflation, the effective rate of return on an investment providing a 6% rate of return is really 2%. And that ignores possible federal, state, and local income taxes which, in some states, could eliminate the return altogether. Given life expectancies, most financial software programs project a 4% drawdown on a portfolio as a means of preserving sufficient income to fund retirement.

Even though in some years there may be a low rate of return, through the magic of compounding, your money will likely grow in value over time. The *earlier* you start, and the sooner you *regularly* save, the more likely that you'll be further ahead in the long term.

Therefore, with this in mind, you should start investing in your 20s, or soon after you obtain your first full-time job. If you have student loans, consider consulting with a financial advisor about whether it is wise to use investable money to pay them off. The decision is likely a function of the assumed rate of investment return versus the interest rate payable on the student loan.

At all ages, you should consider contributing to a 401(k) or other retirement account to the maximum amount allowed, taking into consideration your living expenses. If you take home all of your earnings, it may be difficult to fight the temptation to spend on frivolous items money that could be saved. Over a lifetime, even a small monthly contribution of $50 to $100 can translate into significant savings. And in most cases your employer will match your contribution, up to a certain level.

An Individual Retirement Account ("IRA") is another type of tax-deferred retirement vehicle. An IRA allows you to save and invest money, only paying taxes as the funds are withdrawn. If you're self-employed, or if your employer doesn't provide a 401(k) plan as a benefit, then you should consider investing in an IRA. An IRA is *self-directed*, whereas a 401(k) is *employer-directed*. With an IRA, you have complete discretion as to the choice of investments. With a 401(k), your employer provides you with a menu of available investments from which to choose. Historically, investors have been able to save more money annually through a 401(k) than an IRA. But with either 401(k)s or IRAs, there are limits to the amounts which can be set aside for retirement in any given year.

Remember, future financial freedom is dependent on the exercise of current financial discipline.

Financial Planning in Your Thirties

As you move into your 30s, saving and accumulating money should be the main goal. If possible, you may consider investing in a well-diversified portfolio consisting of securities, bonds, and mutual funds. Picking individual stocks is difficult and risky – purchasing too many shares of an individual stock can be like putting all of your eggs in a single basket. Thus, you may consider investing in *mutual funds* or *exchange traded funds* (ETFs) which typically invest in a broad spectrum of stocks and/or bonds. Instead of owning stock in a handful of companies, you can effectively own a tiny piece of hundreds of companies. This can insulate you from the financial vagaries of an individual company.

While both mutual funds and ETFs invest similarly, there are significant differences.

Mutual funds are pooled investments where your money is combined with that of other investors and actively managed. Mutual funds are attractive because they provide the expertise of a fund manager who researches companies, governments, and agencies and determines the portfolio mix. While there are no individual shareholder transaction costs, there are internal costs for fund management and, in some cases, "load charges" upon either purchase or sale of the fund. By law, most mutual funds must pay out capital gains. Accordingly, even if you do not sell any interest in a mutual fund, you may have to pay taxes every year on your share of the fund's capital gains.

Exchange traded funds trade like stocks but allow you to invest in particular sectors of the economy or the broader market. For example, you can elect to purchase a technology or energy ETF comprised of multiple companies in that industry or sector. If you are not interested in investing in a particular sector, you can purchase an ETF which tracks the market, like the S&P 500 or the Russell 2000. This will likely provide more stable returns because of the diversification across many industries. You only pay taxes if you sell your interest in the fund.

Mutual funds and/or ETFs are often the centerpiece of portfolios because they provide an opportunity for diversification for smaller investors.

A painless way to save even more money is to *reinvest dividends earned from your portfolio.* If possible, you should also try to increase your 401(k) contributions. Through this decade, you may consider adopting more aggressive investment strategies. On the upside, this can enhance your future retirement portfolio. And, if the investments fail to perform as expected, you still have plenty of time to catch up. As with any type of investing, it is important to consult with a qualified financial advisor.

In your 30s, you should attempt to build an emergency savings fund which can cover at least six months of living expenses in the event of unemployment or an inability to work. This need was highlighted during the COVID-19 pandemic of 2020 when approximately 20% of the workforce became temporarily unemployed. Many furloughed workers, who had been living from paycheck to paycheck, were unable to make their next month's mortgage or rent payment. Reliance on aid from unemployment insurance and government-stimulus payments was in many cases insufficient to cover ongoing obligations.

Since none of us can predict when a future crisis may arise, it is sensible and important to recognize the need to plan for unforeseen events.

In the world of retirement planning, bear in mind that cash is not necessarily king. The returns on cash will never keep pace with the taxes paid on earned interest, which, coupled with inflation, erodes the value of a dollar. After you have provided for an emergency living cushion, cash in the bank should be the smallest piece of your investment pie.

At this stage of life, you should also consider purchasing disability insurance – a product designed to pay you a monthly sum should you become unable to work due to illness or other incapacity. The 30s is typically the decade when many people marry and have children. Thus, you may want to consider purchasing life insurance (either a term or whole life policy). At this stage, due to the significant difference in premiums, you may opt for a term life policy to hedge against your unexpected death. In that unlikely event, the policy proceeds can be used to replace your lost income and perhaps pay off an existing mortgage or student debt.

While most people understand the concept of life insurance, they do not recognize the value in paying premiums for disability coverage. However, at many stages of life, temporary or permanent disability is actually more likely than premature death.

Financial Planning in Your Forties

As you move into your 40s, additional factors must be considered. In addition to the strategies you implemented in your 20s and 30s, you may also need to contemplate saving for your children's college tuition and potentially assisting aging parents. You should continue to maximize your savings and schedule annual reviews with your financial advisor who can revise projections based on changed circumstances and goals.

Financial Planning in Your Fifties

All of the prior activities should continue in your 50s and throughout your working years. During this decade, continue to think about any additional expenses that may crop up – such as paying for a child's wedding – that can impact your long-term financial condition. Additionally, there are other considerations and financial planning tools that you should be aware of:

- The 401(k) program allows individuals over 50 to increase annual contributions.

- You may consider rebalancing your investment portfolio to start hedging against risk. As time and compounding are no longer the strong allies that they once were, if you are heavily invested in a particular business sector or company, a significant market downturn in your portfolio may make it difficult for you to recover, and thus adversely affect your long-term financial goals. While your Social Security projections should also be considered, the estimated future benefits should not be absolutely relied upon.

- This may also be the time to become educated about annuities. Despite what you hear in the media, annuities are another investment tool. Conceptually, an annuity functions like a traditional pension plan. Although they have high up-front expenses and future administration costs, the right annuity can be a part of your overall financial plan, providing a guaranteed stream of income and serving as a hedge against riskier investments which may be in your portfolio.

- As you move into your 50s, there is also likely a place for bonds in your portfolio. This is because *fixed income* should be a piece of your portfolio to partially offset the risk of investing in stocks. A bond is a fixed-income investment which represents a loan to either a corporate, governmental, or agency borrower. The bond has a face amount and, in most cases, a guaranteed interest rate with a set maturity date. For example, if you purchase a $10,000 bond paying a 5% coupon (interest) with a maturity date in 20 years, and you hold the bond until maturity, you will receive $500 per year for 20 years ($10,000 in interest), and, upon maturity, the bond issuer will return your initial investment of $10,000. Many people opt not to hold bonds until maturity and decide to sell them during their term. Reasons may include the need for cash or the desire to use the proceeds for alternative investments. But be aware that if you sell a bond before its maturity, due to prevailing interest rates, you may realize more or less than the face amount of the bond. With the exception of government-issued bonds, where the income is tax-free on the federal level (and sometimes on the state and local levels), the income from corporate and agency bonds is fully taxable. Bonds are also often callable, meaning that the issuer can redeem the bond at an earlier date and prematurely pay you the face amount. This could upset your long-term plans. Because it is not always possible to hold the bond until maturity, you may consider investing in either a bond fund or a bond ETF owning a complete portfolio of bonds. This insulates you against the financial vagaries of a particular company, agency, or government. Ratings agencies such as Standard & Poor's, Moody's, and Fitch provide information on the quality of bonds. Typically, the higher the rating, the lower the bond's interest rate.

- This decade is the ideal time to consider obtaining a long-term care insurance policy to fully or partially pay for care in your residence, in an assisted living community, or, if absolutely necessary, in a skilled-nursing facility. It is important to note that premiums are partially dictated by your age and health. So if you wait too long to purchase a policy, your age may make the premiums prohibitive or your health may make obtaining coverage impossible. The cost of round-the-clock care to assist you with your daily living activities is extremely expensive. In the absence of sufficient long-term care insurance and income, you may be forced to spend down your assets and then seek to become eligible for Medicaid benefits. As with Social Security, the continued availability of Medicaid benefits at current levels is uncertain.

Financial Planning in Your Sixties

As you enter and move through your 60s, you hopefully have passed the decades of significant external obligations (e.g., your own student debt, college tuition for children, and mortgage payments). Although there is a shorter timeline, if you have not fully achieved your financial goals, you should probably tighten your belt and maximize your investing.

This is an extremely important time to consult with your financial advisor. Or if you do not have a financial advisor, you should consider retaining one. You may consider moving a portion of your portfolio into a more *conservative asset allocation*. This can partially insulate you from financial shocks which, because of your age, it may be impossible to recover from. In addition, you should start to think about when to trigger the *receipt of Social Security benefits*. The decision must be considered in the context of several factors, including whether you are still earning wages, your overall health, and other sources of income. You should also check your statement of benefits. The longer you defer the receipt of Social Security benefits, the greater the monthly payment. But, in the future, this tried-and-true axiom may be challenged by concepts such as means-testing, which is being considered as a way to prolong the financial viability of the entire Social Security system. So you should never fully rely on the projections of benefits.

Financial Planning in Your Seventies

If you have not already retired, you will likely do so in your early 70s and begin to draw upon your accumulated financial holdings. Federal law dictates that, at age 72, you *must* start to take annual distributions from your retirement accounts. By this time, you have been receiving Social Security benefits for at least two years. If these two sources of income are insufficient to fund your retirement goals, you need to evaluate options. If you have been reinvesting dividends from your investment, you may now elect to have some or all of those dividends paid to you directly.

Even with your best efforts, if financial security remains uncertain, you can consider such actions as either borrowing against the cash value of a whole life insurance policy or surrendering the policy in exchange for a lump sum payment. But, as such a decision will reduce or even eliminate a death benefit, it must be evaluated as a part of your overall estate plan.

You can also consider obtaining a reverse mortgage on your home. Unlike a conventional mortgage requiring monthly payments, the benefit of a reverse mortgage is that the loan is not repaid until the owner vacates the premises or passes away.

There are many tools and strategies to be considered and weighed. Because of such complexity, it can be extremely helpful to obtain retirement planning advice from qualified financial, insurance, and accounting professionals. It helps to collaborate with a team of advisors, including an estate planning attorney, to ensure that your personal and financial goals are realistic and sustainable. Further, your financial plan should be integrated with your estate plan.

In selecting a competent financial advisor, ask for referrals from other trusted advisors, such as attorneys and accountants, and even friends and relatives. You may want to interview several candidates and understand their general investment philosophy and fee structure. Some will charge a percentage of assets under management, and some charge a fee per transaction. Some will offer to design a full financial/retirement plan. Be candid about your risk tolerance and overall objectives.

Financial Planning in Your Eighties, Nineties, and Hundreds

If you have made it into your 80s, 90s, and 100s, then congratulations! Hopefully, you are healthy and living the life in retirement that you hoped and planned for.

Retirement planning requires much thought and attention throughout all the decades of your life. There are numerous questions to consider, such as the right timing of your retirement, where you might want to live or relocate, perhaps even starting a new journey or "second act."

If you thrive by working and cannot conceive of full retirement, then there is no need to stop. In addition to providing supplemental income and additional financial insurance for longevity, ongoing employment can provide mental stimulation, social engagement, and intergenerational interaction. Or, if you were unable to save adequately for retirement, you may be forced to maintain some level of employment. Retirement may include continued employment in your current occupation on a reduced or part-time basis, or providing consulting services as an independent contractor. Many businesses may encourage ongoing service and dedication from long-standing employees with a vast knowledge base and invaluable experience.

There are many non-financial factors which must be considered and weighed when planning for retirement. These include the type of activities you wish to engage in, such as athletics and hobbies. Many people enjoy traveling, as well as participating in educational programs at universities or institutes. Volunteering and community service can make for a purposeful retirement by giving back and contributing your time, talent, and treasure to local or national organizations or causes. With retirement comes the freedom to devote additional time to issues and causes which resonate with you.

For some, retirement may involve a desire, need, or obligation to care for loved ones. You may choose to provide babysitting services for your grandchildren, easing the financial burden for your adult children while reaping the rewards and benefits of time with your family. You may choose to remain close, or move closer, to your loved ones who will ultimately provide or facilitate your care, if and when you need it.

Planning for retirement entails a kaleidoscope of analyses, including emotional, physical, financial, medical, and legal considerations. By creating realistic budgets, adequately funding savings and retirement accounts, following wise investment strategies, and reacting appropriately to economic and market conditions, you have the best chance to fund and enjoy a future that meets your needs and goals.

23 AN ETHICAL WILL: LEAVING YOUR LEGACY TO LOVED ONES

Wendy K. Goidel, Esq.

Typically, when designing an estate plan, the primary objectives are how best to distribute assets and leave a financial legacy to your spouse, children, or other beneficiaries. The discussions center around the distribution of your assets, or your "valuables and principal." However, your tangible assets may not be the greatest value you pass on to your family. That is because there is another legacy which should be considered: the distribution of your intangible assets, or your "values and principles."

In holistic estate and financial planning, this emotional legacy – or the creation of an "ethical will" – collectively refers to imparting your beliefs, values, feelings, and moral philosophies. Legacy planning does not replace estate planning; rather, it can be incorporated into a comprehensive estate and financial plan. The ethical will, while not an essential legal document, is nevertheless emotionally important. While a trust can be designed to protect your assets for your family for generations, it does not provide any written commentary about why you left certain instructions for their distribution.

The best way to ensure that both your financial and emotional legacies are understood and appreciated is to memorialize them in writing. The ethical will becomes the missing piece of a comprehensive and meaningful estate plan.

Rabbi Joshua Stampfer, when interviewed by Marcy Houle, explained the value of an ethical will:

A traditional will, generally speaking, gives directions about disposition of assets. It can include a house, or furniture, or jewelry, whatever. I believe it's very important, however, to sit down and write a will of the principles and ideas you feel are significant in your life – those you hope your children, grandchildren, and great-grandchildren will pursue. It is not a demand. Not at all. Rather, it is your gift to them.

Since the focus of an ethical will is the distribution of *emotional assets*, knowledge of the law is not required and the document is devoid of legal jargon. Unlike the creation of a traditional Will or Living Trust, there are no rules, regulations, or formalities to follow. Because the document you create is not legally enforceable, it does not need to adhere to any format. It does not need to be witnessed, notarized, stapled, or stored in a vault. You do not need to consult with (or pay) an attorney for the creation and execution of the document. *You* are the drafter and the sole source of information. The document you create is unique to you, as it encapsulates your teachings, stories, values, philosophies, and words of wisdom.

Certainly, these are the true treasures you have spent a lifetime collecting, and which require protection. Rather than risking them to loss or misinterpretation upon your death, your life treasures should be recorded and passed down to your heirs. Your document will hopefully document a life well-lived.

The preparation of an ethical will is not novel – in fact, it dates back to ancient times. While the concept has recently become agnostic, it originated in the Jewish religion, dating back about 3,500 years. There are a number of references to ethical wills in both the Old and New Testaments. The oral tradition of an ethical will evolved into a written document in or about the eleventh century.

Preparing an ethical will can seem overwhelming and intimidating. In truth, it is neither. Rather than a chore to be ignored or abhorred, creating it can be embraced as a labor of love to benefit current and future generations.

The key to writing your unique ethical will is taking the necessary time to reflect. Recall key moments of your life and reflect on their importance. Consider the experiences that shaped and impacted your life, both positively and negatively. Think about what those experiences taught you about yourself, others, and even about life itself. Ask yourself how you want to be remembered. Before drafting your document, you may consider the following questions:

- What beliefs, values, morals, or philosophies shaped your personality?
- How did you acquire or develop your beliefs, values, morals, or philosophies?
- What qualities were important to you?
- What were your life goals?
- What philosophies or actions helped you to become successful in your chosen occupation, career, or profession?
- What philosophies did you subscribe to when saving, investing, and spending money?
- What causes did you support or feel passionate about?
- Do you want your children to continue to support the same causes or adopt different causes?
- What do you wish you could have accomplished had you had the time, funds, or opportunity?
- What difficulties did you experience or overcome, what did you learn from them, and how did you turn them into positive philosophies or teachings?
- What do you want your children, grandchildren, and future generations to learn from your life and values?

After outlining your reflections, you should start to create your ethical will. It can take any form including an essay, letter, paper or digital scrapbook, PowerPoint presentation, video, recording, or any combination of media. Ultimately, you will want to create a product that sincerely and thoroughly presents your legacy to those who will read or view it after you die.

While a multimedia presentation may appeal to younger generations, there should still be an accompanying written letter or document. Keep in mind that current technology may not be available in decades to come. Technology changes and can be replaced. But a written letter could endure forever.

Many resources exist for the creation of ethical wills, such as books, workbooks, tools, templates, and websites. As with any important document, when preparing your ethical will, the first draft should never be the last draft. If time permits, put it aside and review it later. Keep writing and editing until you think it adequately communicates your legacy and strikes the right tone. For those who may not be comfortable putting pen to paper, consider asking a relative, friend, or trusted advisor for help.

Notwithstanding the format of your ethical will, it will be used to impart wisdom and inspiration and communicate countless messages to your family. More specifically, it can be used to:

- express love and appreciation for your family members, friends, and colleagues
- preserve and pass on cherished stories and family information
- document your teachings, values, principles, and spiritual beliefs and how you developed them throughout your lifetime
- share your life's lessons
- share anecdotes about your own life which may help your family to appreciate your struggles, challenges, and/or the personal and professional choices you made
- express any regrets or requests for forgiveness (if necessary). You can also forgive friends, relatives, or business colleagues for their transgressions toward you or others
- provide warnings or cautionary tales
- share your hopes and aspirations for your family

In *Words from the Heart: A Practical Guide to Writing an Ethical Will* (2015), E. L. Weiner suggests that ethical wills be written from the heart and contain feelings and anecdotes from the HEART: H = hopes for the future; E = experiences in life; A = appreciation; R = religion, spirituality, and core beliefs; T = treasures.

When creating your ethical will, try thinking about the five parts of this acronym. Share your unique voice; be genuine and maintain authenticity. The letter should represent you and your values.

Remember, these are the intangible lessons which, if not documented and shared, will be lost forever.

Whether your life was exciting or simple matters little. Also irrelevant is where you fall on the socioeconomic spectrum. Never think that, because you did not win awards or achieve wealth or fame during your education, career, or life, your story is unimportant. Instead, it is undoubtedly of great value to those you love. If you have always been reluctant to share anecdotes about your family history and stories from your life, there is a good likelihood that your children or other relatives will yearn to hear them when you are gone. Your letter will provide an indelible and everlasting legacy for your family.

While many people write their ethical wills toward the latter part of their lives, it need not be done as last-minute death-bed planning. It can be written at any stage of life or over many years; it can be a work in progress spanning many decades. Letters can be written before or after life cycle events, such as marriage, the birth of a child, a significant illness, or the passing of a loved one.

For example, some parents write a letter to each of their children on their birthdays, documenting the highlights of that year and their hopes and dreams for the next year. For others, starting to write an ethical will at a younger age may help them make certain choices so their lives become rich with purpose, intention, and meaning.

Remember, there is no right or wrong way to write an ethical will. Some choose to write one overarching ethical will to be shared with the entire family. Others prefer separate letters containing personal messages, feelings, inspiration, and information for specific family members.

For your ethical will to act as the vehicle through which you leave your emotional legacy, your family *needs to know it exists*. You may even opt to share your ethical will with your family during your lifetime, rather than after you die. Your ethical will can be added to your estate planning portfolio or stored with your legal documents, along with instructions about who can see it and when. If you choose not to wait until your death for its disclosure, you can allow your family to read or view it during your lifetime with or without you present. Sharing the contents while you are still alive can provide inspiration or even help your family to repair relationships and grow closer.

A well-designed and well-written ethical will can become the gift that keeps on giving. Your financial assets are easily quantifiable and can be quickly spent. While the value of the intangible contents of your ethical will is impossible to quantify, it will last for generations to come.

24 YOU'VE BECOME A CAREGIVER

Now What?

Elizabeth Eckstrom, MD, MPH, MACP

Caregiving is hard work, and caregivers often feel totally isolated in their role. But you are not alone. In fact, recent statistics show that over 66 million people in the US are caring for someone – a parent, spouse, child, family member, or friend. With the tremendous growth of people over age 65 – 10,000 people a day cross that marker in the US alone – it is expected that in the next 20 years nearly every middle-aged person will be caregiving for someone.

Most people become caregivers because they love the one they are caring for, and many have no other option. Yet no matter how and when they step into the role, few have any idea what lies ahead. Caregiving entails a broad scope of duties that for many caregivers are piled on an already full plate. They take the one they care for to visit their doctors, schedule necessary appointments, maybe manage a variety of medications, and in general help them navigate a fragmented healthcare / health insurance system. As well, they may need to help out with housework and make sure their care partner is eating properly.

All of this takes a toll, mentally and physically. Caregivers quickly discover there is no clear charted course for them, and it is a job for which few have had any previous training. This is why it's important to recognize that there is another side of caregiving most of us don't think about, but which is critically important over the long term:While we focus our attention on the one who needs our assistance, we need also to *care for ourselves*.

I regularly see family caregivers suffer. They feel it is selfish to complain about their situation when they see themselves as being much better off than the one who needs their assistance. It's easy to think that we "should" be able to do it all: give our care partner the emotional support they truly need, hold down our job, take care of other family members, and simply manage to add these new responsibilities into the mix along with everything else.

Orchestrating all these competing priorities leaves caregivers feeling exhausted, lonely and anxious, cut off from friends, and turning to the Internet for help because they don't know where else to turn. Then they feel guilty for all those feelings, because they aren't the ones who are supposed to need help.

But this is the huge misconception. Caregivers *do* need help. They need to learn that it is okay to feel guilty, tired, sad, and angry. That's *normal*. They need to understand that caregiving is a *two-way relationship*. Both sides need replenishment and reinforcement. Maintaining our own health and happiness and other relationships is crucial to the one doing the caregiving. The big question is how do we do that amidst all of the challenges?

I tell my patients to think of these "Seven Core Strategies" that can provide the support and renewal caregivers need throughout their journey. Since caregiving needs rarely go down and usually go up, it's important to start planning early.

1 Look For Outside Help

At the onset, research what community resources are available. Admittedly, this is a big task and takes a lot of time to pursue, so give yourself permission to take all the time you need. Check out state-sponsored Area Agencies on Aging, the Alzheimer's Association, the local senior center, and other community organizations. Ask your doctor for links to services. Many faith communities give assistance. Some have networks of drivers to assist those who no longer drive. Others offer help getting family members to appointments. Caregiving needs change over time, so keep a broad list of resources and follow good leads that professionals give you.

2   Find a Support Group

Not all caregivers will choose this option, but for many who do, the benefits can be immeasurable. Whether you are a child caring for a mother with Alzheimer Dementia, a spouse tending to a husband with Parkinson Disease, or a parent dealing with a child with special needs, belonging to a support group can bring new friends and associations into your life who will understand what you are going through and provide ideas for coping. It is a relief to be with people who "get it," and seeing others who have a more difficult situation than you have can help put your own trials in perspective.

3   Figure Out a Self-Care Plan, and Do It

What provides *you* with joy and refreshment? Gardening, walking, cycling, or running? Playing the piano, listening to music, seeing friends for lunch, going to spiritual services? The important thing is to *put these things on a calendar.* It might seem crazy, but if you like to play the piano, put piano on your calendar every day from 4.30 to 5 p.m., or whenever could be a good break time for you. And then, check that calendar. See if you are following these self-care stratagems. If you find you're skipping them because life is too hectic, reevaluate how you might find that time for yourself. The critical point is to *plan and develop a strategy* that works for you, and that you can follow its progress on your calendar.

4   If At All Possible, Enlist Some Outside Help for Your Care Partner's Physical Needs

While taking care of your care partner's physical needs is important, other people can step in and help with these tasks. But perhaps no one can provide the emotional support and love that *you* can. This is something to be protected and fostered. If you are worn out from all the physical demands, you won't have energy left over to supply this most valued task. Whenever you can, get assistance with physical needs so that you can reserve your energy for the important emotional tasks.

5 Maintain Your Own Health

It's particularly easy to neglect yourself when your focus is completely on someone else. That's why it is essential to be on the lookout to see if your own health might be suffering. Experiencing symptoms such as trouble sleeping, being overly fatigued, becoming depressed, and developing bodily aches or abdominal problems are all red flags. This is when you should talk to *your* doctor, and receive the care *you* need.

6 Make Time to Reflect on Your Situation

This is a strategy most of us don't think about, partly because we feel we don't have enough time, but also because it's one of the more difficult things to do. Often it helps to keep a journal of your feelings. Recognize that none of your feelings are "bad." There will be times when you'll feel sorry for yourself and wonder "Why me?" And times when you wish you could just go back to "the way things were before." You will grieve that your care partner "isn't the same." There will even be days when you just wish your care partner would die and it could all be over. This is normal. It is all part of a *grieving process*. By thinking about these feelings consciously and letting them see the light of day, you will face them for what they are: emotions of sadness, as well as indications that you need some respite time for yourself. By reflecting, you can also find the positives that remain. You can pride yourself on how you are handling the tough situation. You will be able to help others in similar situations of caregiving. For you are not alone. Thousands are going through the same things you are. It can help to know that there is a wide network out there traveling through similar journeys.

7 Find Your Team

This simple strategy may be the most essential of all. And it's one to consider at the very beginning of your new life as a caregiver. Your work is hard; you will need to share the load. Consider those you can turn to when life gets out of balance and you are exhausted, frightened, and need someone to lean on. Who are they? Who could you call at midnight, or when yet another crisis comes up? They may include a spouse, a neighbor or close friend, a counselor or minister, a sister, brother, or cousin. Don't forget the Alzheimer Association, which has a 24-hour phone line to help with crises. The important thing is that you know they will be there for you when you need them. They are your *team*. And the sooner you can identify them the better, because not sharing the hard parts of your life with someone you trust will only become more difficult as time goes on. Relationships are what will help when the going gets tough. Your team can be there at the toughest times. And for those who have gone through this, they will say "That's what life's all about."

Caregiving is a hard job, but it is also a "heart" job. After it is over, the greatest comfort you can know is that you have cared, you have invested yourself, and you have loved.

25 SO MANY LIVING ARRANGEMENTS

Which One Is for You?

Elizabeth Eckstrom, MD, MPH, MACP

There is no place like home.

The thing is, home may have different definitions depending on a host of factors – one's culture, means, availability, requirements, preferences, needs, functions.

Now add to that a new element: aging.

There are so many different options for living arrangements as we age that most of us would have difficulty naming them or defining what they mean. For that reason, and others, we tend to put off thinking about them. Most of us like the idea of "aging in place," yet that might not be a possibility as we grow older, might not be our preference, and might not be best for our health. At the other end of the spectrum is the dreaded alternative in many people's minds: a nursing home.

When all we know are these two "bookend" selections for housing – our family home and a nursing home – it's easy to put off any kind of planning for the future. But there are many other possibilities available. That's why understanding the wide variety of opportunities is a good idea. If there comes a time when you aren't able to remain in your home, you want to have some options already thought out, which is the best way to avoid an emergency placement in a nursing home. This chapter is heavily slanted to options available in the US, and I encourage people in other countries to look into your own options.

In considering the choices, think about your needs, now and in the future. How can you remain socially engaged and not isolated? What can you afford? Consider location – near family? With family? What about health issues over time? What activities are important to you? What things do you value the most?

More and more diverse living arrangements are becoming available all the time, and many of the models are new and highly creative. Options fall into eleven major living categories. Understanding what they are helps remove some of our hesitation in thinking about them, and allows us to consider what might be a possibility in our future.

Aging in Place This is staying in your current living situation. If this is your goal, make the modifications you will need *before* you need them. This will likely include putting grab bars in the bathroom, adding wheelchair ramps, putting lights in dark corners, removing throw rugs to prevent falls, and figuring out how to live on the ground floor if your house has more than one level. Evaluate how to meet your transportation needs once you are no longer driving (do NOT assume you will drive until you die – men have to stop driving an average of 7 years before they die, and women have to stop driving an average of 10 years before they die). Figure out how you will meet your caregiving needs.

Nearly everyone needs some assistance before they die, whether with finances, shopping, and cleaning, or with more basic tasks like bathing, dressing, and using the toilet. Some people will require assistance 24/7 – especially if they develop dementia. Home care costs add up quickly if your care needs are high, and are not affordable for most older people. And some people feel they must stay in their home no matter what. They then discover they can't get out and only have visitors every week or two, leading to terrible social isolation. Services such as Meals on Wheels and free transportation to local community centers can help reduce isolation, but many people who stay in their home become very isolated. They are utterly surprised to feel they have a wonderful new life in front of them when they finally "give in" and move to assisted living or some other supportive environment.

Aging in Place living is evolving. Some older adults might bring in a renter to offset costs and provide companionship and help around the house. Others may build an "Accessory Dwelling Unit" next to their larger home to house a renter or family member or caregiver. Some move from the family home into a smaller, more accessible house or apartment to make it easier to remain independent.

Villages Founded in Boston in 2002, this is another model, akin to Aging in Place but with something special added. It is "neighbors-helping-neighbors" and is becoming very popular all across the nation. Villages is a membership-based community with a reasonable sliding-scale membership fee, and operates with paid staff and volunteers who can assist members with a myriad of services – transportation, simple home repairs, grocery shopping. Everyone is encouraged to volunteer, and to look out for one another.

Intergenerational Housing These innovative living options benefit both older persons and children, twining them together into a community. They are often located in apartment buildings, generally affordable, and can provide a stable "home" for low-income senior citizens connecting with foster youth, bringing an intentional sense of stability and mentorship.

EngAGE Senior Arts Colonies Developed by aging expert Tim Carpenter, EngAge is a non-profit organization that offers seniors communities that are focused on wellness, the arts, intergenerational opportunities, and life-long learning. These are housing units that serve low- and moderate-income seniors, and consist of apartments united around an arts-themed community. Started in Burbank, California, it is a model that is taking off in other parts of the country.

Green House Model of Care Geriatrician Bill Thomas revolutionized the idea of nursing homes with the "Green House" model. These living arrangements lodge residents who need significant care, but the tastefully decorated, innovative rooms don't feel anything like a hospital or traditional nursing home. Instead, these residences strike a balance between group living with support staff and independent rooms, woven with community living spaces. Together, they make long-term care feel like, as many residents say, they are living in a "home."

Continuing-Care Retirement Communities (CCRCs) These communities, which tend to be the highest-end and most expensive places, include different housing options, all within a framework of a larger residential setting. CCRCs generally offer numerous social activities and services; some might have onsite beauty shops and entertainment venues. As residents' health needs change, they allow for care transitions – the ability to move from one level of care to another – from independent apartment living to assisted living, memory care, and skilled nursing.

Age-Restricted Communities These can include homes, neighborhoods, condominiums, and apartments that generally don't have care services but are designed to accommodate people usually at least 55 and older. "Age-Restricted Communities" offer age-delineated social opportunities and activities that may include sports that residents can engage in, golf courses, a gym, or pool. Houses, townhouses, or other apartments are available to own or rent, depending on the requisites of the individual community.

Assisted Living These living arrangements provide meals, housekeeping, recreational activities, and transportation to and from appointments. Services vary widely between assisted living facilities, so it is important to learn what is offered at the facility you are interested in. Some have nursing staff on a limited basis for medical assistance, but most of them still require you to have a fair degree of independence. If you need assistance with medications, bathing, or other daily tasks, they will most certainly charge additional fees for those services.

Adult Foster Homes For seniors with significant care needs, such as needing assistance with bathing and dressing, adult foster homes (I like to call them "Adult Family Homes") can be a great option. They are smaller in size, with up to five residents who each have their own bedrooms but share a communal living and dining room. They provide meals, transportation to doctors' offices,

and some even manage people who are on ventilators permanently. They offer a home-like environment for older adults who
require substantial assistance, usually with staff who are as dedicated to providing that care as family members would be. I cannot
speak highly enough of our local adult family homes. They are
run by some of the most skilled, caring, and loving people in our
community.

Memory Care Facilities These residences are specifically
designed for people with dementia. They have a higher number
of staff specially trained to care for people with Alzheimer Disease
and other forms of dementia. They include security features to
help keep residents safe inside the facility.

Nursing Homes These are for older adults who have complex
medical issues and need assistance with nearly all basic activities.
They are licensed and regulated by state agencies, and provide 24-
hour supervision. Nursing home residents can be supported by
speech, occupational, and physical therapists to help them manage activities of daily living. Attributes and quality can vary tremendously among these facilities. As with any selection you
choose, *do your homework.*

Most of us prefer to remain independent as we age. But
most of us need assistance at some point. I always tell my
patients: "Hope for the best, but plan for the worst." Where we
live is one of the most important considerations as we age. If
you have a daughter or son who can move in and care for you
24 hours a day, consider yourself lucky. Virtually no one
has that anymore, so we have to prepare for our future care
needs.

Long-term care insurance can help people afford home and
alternative options, especially if you were foresighted enough
to get it 20 or 30 years ago. If your resources are scarce, talk
with a financial planner to figure out what options are available to you, and don't wait too long to implement them.

I cannot tell you how many patients I have had who lived in
their own home (even though I encouraged them to move) after
they couldn't drive anymore and became very socially isolated,
depressed, deconditioned, and cognitively impaired. When they

finally moved to assisted living, a CCRC, or an adult family home, they made new friends, were able to go out to events again, and had their care needs met. Nearly everyone has told me "I should have listened to you and made this move years ago!"

26 DO THIS ONE SIMPLE THING TO ADD 7.5 YEARS TO YOUR LIFE!

Elizabeth Eckstrom, MD, MPH, MACP

There are many types of prejudices, but only one that is universal to *all* people if they live long enough. It applies to everyone, regardless of skin color, religion, gender, or all the other ways we too often categorize people. For those who are directly suffering from it, it can significantly reduce their well-being and even their life expectancy.

What is this prejudgment that is pervasive throughout society, hurts over 1 billion people worldwide, yet millions of us partake in it and even find it socially acceptable?

Ageism.

Ageism is the stereotyping, inequity, exclusion, and discrimination of people on the basis of their age. At the same time the older population is growing rapidly – over 2 billion people will be over 60 by 2050 – ageism is rampant, both overtly and insidiously. If you, as a younger person, have ever passed over an older adult, you are perpetuating a preconception that will come back to haunt you when you are older. Or, as Josh Kornbluth starkly put it in his Citizen Brain series, "If we have bad thoughts about older people, we are also being biased against our *future self.*"

If you have been fortunate to have lived a life of privilege, you will *not* be immune. Even people who have enormously successful careers, families, and networks grow old; they will lose hearing and sight, and find themselves passed over. As Marcy discovered with her parents' trajectory – when very old, they became just a "head in the bed." Ageism takes many forms: from "acceptable" ones of being the brunt of "geezer" jokes to feeling invisible to society and even shunned.

An astounding *80%* of older adults report ageism has impacted their lives. Many older people express that people just *assume* they have memory or physical impairments due to their age. One-third report being ignored or not taken seriously because they are old. Over half disclose they have been recipients of jokes that poke fun at older people.

Even more serious, health professionals may assess older people incorrectly – diagnosing problems such as cognitive impairment or psychological disorders as the result of their *age* rather than the real culprits: too many drugs – some unsafe – being prescribed; undiagnosed medical problems; substance use disorders.

Consequences of this discrimination can be severe. Besides suffering mental and physical health issues that go undiagnosed, those who suffer from ageism have lower life expectancy. Negative self-perceptions of aging involve reduced self-efficacy, with direct effects on depression. Biases can discourage older people from freely participating in work or recreational activities and can contribute to social isolation, limiting their ability to make a positive contribution to the collective whole, and perpetuating fear of aging in all individuals.

A 2020 comprehensive global research report of 7 million participants worldwide – individuals from 45 countries, 11 health domains, and lasting 25 years – showed that ageism led to *worse health outcomes in 95% of the studies*. Evidence of ageism was found across age, sex, and race/ethnicity of subjects.

Is there anything we can do to eradicate ageism and prevent ourselves from succumbing to it when we are old? Yes. The first step is recognizing we have a *systemic problem* and it is teeming around the world. The second is realizing that *our own anxiety about aging itself* exacerbates the problem and tends to lead to ageism. The third is for us to work to develop a positive attitude toward older persons and our own aging. When we do, it not only helps protect us from future injustices, but does something more: *positive feelings about aging can actually add years to our lives.*

Seven and a half years, to be exact.

A large study led by Yale University's Professor Becca Levy, Ph.D., documented that those who held more positive self-perceptions of aging lived 7.5 years longer. Can you think of anything else that gives you that much added longevity? People who think positively about aging have improved mental health, memory, and balance compared to those who don't. They are more likely to recover from disability than those who believe negative age stereotypes. Embracing positive beliefs about aging can help protect against dementia, even among elders with high-risk genes.

Holding negative self-perceptions on aging can do just the opposite. Such pessimistic sensibilities contribute to worse memory and to feelings of worthlessness. What are these impressions? Thinking of living long as a loss. Believing that aging inevitably leads to disability and frailty. That growing old will rob us of our creativity and ability to contribute to work, our communities, and society. That after a certain age (fill in the blank), you will have made all the contributions you will ever make, and will have no worth after that.

These perceptions not only are untrue, they make us fearful about aging. They add to the discrimination that many older people experience. How much better to learn all you can about aging well (as you are doing by reading this book!) and blasting the stereotypes!

You met Lucille, the 101-year-old calligrapher earlier in this book. She has made herself and others happy all her life, and has not become "invisible" as she has aged! Like countless older people, she repudiates the notion that the "only thing worse than old age is death." She continues to contribute to society and adds joy to many people's lives.

I can't help sharing an email she sent to Marcy, while deep in the COVID-19 pandemic:

Marcy, I just had my 100th birthday. I had thought that there was no way there could be much of a celebration during COVID, and that was fine – there would be next year. But people are finding new ways to do the events that we want to observe together.

For my birthday, my church had an amazing drive-by, with two fire trucks in the procession, with signs, balloons and horns honking, while neighbors and my son and daughter-in-law joined me out front. There was a basket of 150 cards (the family had tried for 100). There were six Zoom/Portal calls that put me in touch with friends and family all over, plus a call from Italy and one from Australia.

So I really had a birthday that couldn't be surpassed, wouldn't you say?

Yes, I agree. And following Lucille's lead, I encourage everyone to fight aging discrimination, develop a positive attitude about aging – in society and in yourself – and add 7.5 years to your life!

Action Items to Reduce Ageism in Yourself

- Find ways to stay positive about age and increase lifespan. Consider aging a privilege and an honor; find ways to reframe aging.
- Never consider a health or mental problem the result of "normal aging." Find a healthcare provider that does not dismiss problems as "normal aging"; preferably find a geriatrician or a primary care physician that focuses on older adults!
- Do not socially isolate. Continue to make friends and be a part of society. Make younger friends so they don't die before you.
- Educate yourself on aging (you are already doing that as you read this!) and learn the misconceptions to guard against.
- Get your kids to spend time with grandparents or volunteer with older adults so that they can experience the positive sides of aging.

PART IV
Caring For Your Soul

PART IV

Caring For Your Soul

The past is past and this is where I am now. I am determined to be happy wherever I am.

Mary Hughes,
age 90

27 I DON'T WANT TO GO DOWNSTAIRS!

Marcy Cottrell Houle

The picture on the table catches my attention the moment I enter the office. It is of an older woman with short cropped, white hair, oval face, a generous smile and arm lifted as if waving to a crowd. She looks so happy I can't help smiling back.

"That's Mary," says Susan, "my mother. Just a few years after that picture was taken she died a peaceful death at 92. She was on hospice then, and had been for over 2½ years."

This vital-looking, 90-year old woman on hospice?

"In 2½ years, my mother suffered 3 heart attacks, several mini-strokes, a major stroke, a 1½ inch laceration of her scalp, severe angina episodes at least once a week, and a broken ankle. The amazing thing is, not only was she never admitted, she never set foot in a hospital!"

Susan has my attention now. I think of the thousands of older persons, including my mother, who spent nearly every other weekend in the hospital with one "event" after another, or so it seemed. I wished I could have kept my mother from that fate. What magic did this woman have?

"My mother had a very positive attitude, and a wonderful primary care physician, who had been with her for over 20 years. And she had a very good ending, one I think most people want to have," says Susan. "As much as possible, she planned for it, accepting the risks. She believed in palliative care and was not afraid of death. Her main wish was to keep away from the hospital, and to be treated in place. And most of all, to not go downstairs."

"Not go downstairs?"

"Downstairs was where the skilled nursing was," Susan explains. "She saw, over and over, her friends who would go downstairs never came upstairs again. Mary loved her room at the Assisted Living community where she lived for 3 years. Before that she had lived in Independent Living for 10 years. She raised colorful, blooming orchids and kept them in her room. She loved that she had three windows letting in lots of light, and friends down the hall who would come to see her. Many were old and frail, as she was, but they lived close enough that they could visit. She missed them when they went downstairs. That's why she always told anyone who came to see her, 'I'm better now', no matter what had happened the day before ... or just an hour ago!"

Regarding the merry photograph once more, I settle back in my chair, curious to learn more about this woman. But I am baffled. When people have heart attacks, accidents, or mini-strokes, don't they need to go to the hospital? What about when people get things like pneumonia?

"Let me be a bit clearer," Susan says, reading my mind. "My mother had incurable heart problems. Three years before she died, she did go to the hospital to get a pacemaker. But that was the last time she ever went. She was one to chart her own course. After her pacemaker, she was put on hospice because of her severe inoperable heart disease. She made the decision that, if she died, she wanted to die in place and not have extraordinary measures."

"And she had *you*," I say. Mary had a daughter. An advocate.

"Yes, she was lucky to have me, that is true. And she had a physician she loved and trusted. But she would have made the same decisions, regardless. The measures she took any older person could do. My mother's gift is how she looked at death. She faced it head on. She would say, in a matter-of-fact manner, about her blocked coronary arteries: 'Well, they can't fix it.' Plus, she did lots of advance planning for the kind of end-of-life journey she wanted. She was all for palliative care and hospice, when needed. And Mary was the first person to have her POLST form in the new statewide Registry."

Susan beams with a smile much like her mother's. I suspect she has also inherited Mary's good nature, dynamic will, and determination to help others. Already Susan has made the world

a better place, and given countless individuals relief and assur-
ance that their health wishes will be heard and honored.

Dr. Susan Tolle, an internal medicine physician at Oregon
Health & Science University and Director of OHSU's Center for
Ethics in Health Care, is a founding developer of the POLST program. POLST, standing for Portable Orders for Life-Sustaining
Treatment, has changed the way thousands of people have died.
It is now used by millions all across the United States and in at
least 20 other countries. Patients with a serious illness or frailty
can ask their healthcare provider to specify medical orders on
a POLST form (POLST has slightly different names in some states)
for what kinds of treatment they wish to have if they are found in
an emergency situation. These accompany one's advance directive and turn a person's wishes into a provider order that must be
followed. They are designed to be fluid between all providers
throughout a health calamity – adhered to by paramedics,
EMTs, fire departments – often first on the scene – and also emergency departments, hospitals, and nursing homes.

POLSTs are *medical* forms that travel with you on paper or in
your electronic health record. Their beauty is that, when clinicians
open up your medical record, they can readily see your POLST
form. These orders have kept many thousands of patients from
spending miserable last days on earth tethered to a ventilator or
feeding tubes in the ICU.

Susan looks thoughtful. "When I started practicing, there were
so many people I was seeing in the hospital near the end of their
lives and spending too much time in the ICU when that is not
where they wanted to be, and it troubled me deeply. Patients
would come in with advanced dementia and pneumonia and be
put on ventilators and feeding tubes because no one could find
any records of their wishes for end-of-life care. Most of the patients
died. And they were often delusional at the end and in restraints.
That's what led me to create the POLST program. And of course,
there was my mother."

"Your mother?"

"Mary was involved with POLST from the beginning. She was
a microbiologist by training, and Supervisor for the Pediatric

Microbiology Laboratory at OHSU. She co-authored research papers, taught a generation of physicians, and worked to save the lives of very sick babies. She knew that she didn't want a frantic, sad, end of life, with extraordinary measures enacted during an emergency or mechanical treatments that had little chance of extending her life in any good way. She was a true believer when it came to POLST."

Susan laughs. "Her infectious enthusiasm got others to join the faith. My mother and her doctor signed the very first form for the registry – before there even *was* a registry – so we could make a movie about it and get the registry funded. Then she got many of the people at her community to sign, and soon the entire facility was behind it! Today, almost every state has a developing or functional POLST program. We are now working with community health workers in rural areas and with patients speaking different languages. My mother's advocacy for the program helped spearhead all of this. She was a pioneer."

Susan turns to her mother's vivacious picture. "In a way, it helped chart her own destiny several years later. It provided a planned final chapter of her life, where she could make choices that enabled her to retain independence and control for as long as possible. She chose this very picture to go with the obituary, which she wrote herself, several years before she died! What kind of individual writes her own obituary and then picks a picture of herself waving goodbye?"

"A forthright one; a vigorous one; a planner!" I reply, laughing too, feeling impressed. I still must fight the urge to wave back at the photograph.

"We all were aware what our mother wanted; we were all on the same page before the end. We knew if she ever got dementia (which, thankfully, she didn't) she didn't want a feeding tube or ventilator. She understood the value of communication and advance planning, and not waiting for one giant event to force your hand. It is a trajectory. Good preparation leads to a rewarding death that a family can feel peaceful about."

The thought is arresting. I had heard many unfortunate stories of families who were not at peace with their loved one's death, because either there were no instructions on what to do in an emergency, or not all family members were incorporated in the process. For years, they second-guessed whether the right thing was done. Life's darkest moment was left dark for them.

This same reasoning also sometimes pertains to first responders who come to the scene, finding an older person without a heartbeat. Studies show only 1–3% of older people found in this condition can be resuscitated. Responders' scope of practice, however, compels them to try CPR if there are no instructions available, even though they know, almost invariably, that the patient will die. Responders often are left feeling unsettled.

"Tell me more about the trajectory," I ask, understanding the need for planning, but wondering how many people, myself included, want to begin preparing early for their death.

"It's really not just about planning," Susan explains, "it's about retaining control of your life. The first part is to recognize it's a step-by-step process. The second is to not fear death. Most of the steps come gradually, and there can be lots of good times in-between, even if at first they may not seem so. For Mary, the first thing was having to give up driving. No one wants to do that! But her eyesight was diminishing. Then she began having trouble with her heart. She had wide swings in her blood pressure, which led to little strokes, which led to falls. She realized it would be dangerous to stay alone in her home, where she could have an event, fall, and get really hurt.

"*That* was a hard decision," Susan continues. "To move from her home. And it didn't come without pain. But she did accede to it. When she turned 80, because of health concerns, she moved to a continuing-care retirement community that offers Independent Living and more intensive care if needed. What surprised her most? She loved it!"

Mary obviously did, evidenced from her shining countenance in other photographs Susan shows me.

"She had already been living alone for a year. I don't think she realized how lonely she was! In her new living arrangement, she returned to being social. She loved playing Scrabble. She was a tremendous gardener, and had been a long-time member of the Clematis Society, who now transplanted 80 clematis to the grounds! She lived in Independent Living for 10 years, making close friends, eating with them, having intellectual stimulation.

"I saw first-hand the value of socialization," Susan says. "Another added benefit, it improved her mental functioning. For 10 years after the move, she was conducting her own business better than she had 6 months before her move! Without the community, she wouldn't have had the fun. She told me 'Susan, it's like living in a college dorm only you have money!'"

Susan passes on one of her mother's secrets for successful aging. *Mary didn't look back.* She believed in the value of keeping her sights on what lay ahead, not behind.

It's easy to always be looking in the rear-view mirror, Susan says. It can seem like you are losing more than you are gaining. But that's when Mary stepped out. She did not drive forward by looking in the rear-view mirror. She kept her eyes focused ahead, on what was compelling her, drawing her forth – those things she still had and enjoyed and that brought meaning and a sense of fulfillment to her life.

This became even more evident after she had fainted and needed surgery for an ailing heart, Susan says. During an operation to implant a pacemaker, doctors observed that the blood flow to every part of her heart muscle was seriously compromised. Upon recovery, they admitted Mary to hospice, judging that a major cardiac event would happen at any time and that she needed hospice to control her episodes of severe cardiac pain.

"But my mother, even in her increasing frailty, kept her joy and sparkle," Susan says. "She moved into the Assisted Living portion of the facility and liked that, too. She always said, '*I am determined to be happy wherever I am.*' "

I liked her spunk. Mary Hughes gave evidence that we do have some control over our thoughts and feelings, even when we go through difficult circumstances. And Mary did not die. As Susan relates, her mother lived for 3 more years, during that time surviving more than 25 different events that would have qualified her to go to the hospital. Each time, though, she refused to go, and managed with creative solutions.

"My mother was tenacious. Her conversation changed from '*if* I die' to '*when* I die.' She would say, 'The past is past and this is where I am now.'"

With that spirit, when walking became more difficult for her because of her heart, Mary transitioned to using an electric scooter, without complaint.

"She used that scooter for 3½ years. She tootled everywhere with it. She'd ride it to Scrabble games, to the garden, to see her friends. Our problem was, we were always having to 'negotiate' with her to use only the *very lowest* speed! She also used her scooter," Susan sighs, "to force open doors."

Mary loved spending time outdoors in the facility's garden. Double doors stood at the entrance. As her strength diminished and the weight of the doors grew too heavy for her to manage, she had figured out how to maneuver through them successfully. Revving up her scooter, she would use its momentum to plow the doors open, allowing her to freely access the flower garden. One day, though, Mary failed to notice a large, ceramic pot tipped over on the other side of the entrance. She pushed through the doors, but crashed into the flower pot and fell into the garden. Somehow, she righted herself, and climbed back aboard her scooter. She told no one about her accident. She hurried on to have dinner with her friends as planned, and did not say a word about it to them.

That night, though, Susan received a call.

"Your mother can't stand," the nurse said anxiously over the phone. "Something is wrong with her ankle. She can't bear any weight at all."

Susan went directly over. Mary was in bed, with her foot outside the covers. She was wearing the little ankle brace she always used, because of an unstable ligament. A little later, a mobile X-ray team came to the room.

Mary's ankle was broken.

"When I told my mother the news, she said, 'Well, that's too bad.' I said, 'We need to go to the hospital.' She said, 'I will *not* go to the hospital.' Exasperated, I replied, 'Then what do you propose we do? If you don't get it fixed, you will never walk again!' 'Then *find a new plan'* she told me, but next gave a smile that she gave to everyone who helped her.

"That's why everyone loved her," Susan continues, shaking her head. "After every one of these roller-coaster rides with her health, she would somehow come back. She would tell everyone who helped her, 'Thank you, Sweetheart.' She would be placed on home hospice, which people in the US can qualify for if they are deemed to have 6 months or less to live, and when it looked like she was too stable and should be taken off it, she would have another event, and be recertified. With her serious heart events, nurses would be almost certain she was dying, but she always came back to life. One day while at work, I got a call with a question from hospice.

"Is it possible," they asked, "that your mother is immortal?"

Immortal or not, Mary *did* walk again. A technician was called in who supplied boots for patients after surgery. He found one that would fit over her other ankle support. It was a peculiar contraption – boot-over-a-boot – but it worked and kept her pain free and walking.

"Actually, it was a very smart answer to the problem," Susan agrees. "If my mother had had surgery, she would have been non-weight bearing for six weeks. Considering her frailty, she would probably never have walked again. Her wonderful primary care doctor agreed that keeping my mother out of the hospital was the wisest thing we could do for her, and it allowed my mother more years of quality of life."

Birthdays and holiday festivities always enriched Mary's life, but one event stood out above the rest, Susan discloses. It became a tradition. Every Christmas Eve, Mary would host dinner for her family in a private dining room at the facility. She loved caroling with her family all joining in, her children and grandchildren coming from near and far. For 13 years, Mary reserved the room, paid for it in advance, and treasured the joyous time they could all be together.

Three years ago, though, was different.

"Two weeks before Christmas, my mother had another 'incident,'" Susan recounts, "but this time a major stroke. It rendered her unable to leave her room. She was still cognizant but desperately weak, yet once again refused to go to the hospital."

Mary remained determined, however, that the cherished event go on.

"Everyone knew she didn't have much time. Instead of gathering in the dining room, that night the whole family came up to her room. For four hours we sang Christmas carols, laughing through all our tears. Every member of her family was there, as well as the aides, crying because they too loved her! My mother was on oxygen, yet still to each one of us she would open her eyes and say, 'Sweetheart, I'm so glad to see you.'

"Finally, after midnight, my mother fell asleep. We all stayed close to her, my sister holding her hand. It was just as Mary had planned all along – she got everything she wanted; she had done everything she'd set out to do. There was nothing left to do. She died peacefully in the wee hours of Christmas morning," Susan says softly, "at dawn, surrounded by love, still holding my sister's hand, in a room filled with flowers."

... A room with morning light shining through three large windows, tinging with color the glorious orchids she loved –

Upstairs.

28 HOW NOT TO BE AFRAID OF DYING AND ENSURE THAT YOUR FAMILY REMEMBERS YOUR DEATH AS A PEACEFUL ONE

Elizabeth Eckstrom, MD, MPH, MACP

Wow. I have read the story of Susan's mom many times now and I cry every time. To hear Susan describe all the accidents, crises, frailty, and hospice interactions in such a positive light, and have such peace and joy in describing Mary's death, is pretty amazing. Where is the fear of dying? Where is the family discord about respecting her wishes? Where is the remorse over not "doing enough" medically? Not necessary. Mary and her entire family had many honest, blunt, pragmatic conversations that allowed Susan to guide the family in ensuring that Mary's wishes were met. And Mary faced her own declining health with realism, joy in what she had, and the same skill she brought to her finances: impeccable planning. How can we all emulate this wonderful approach to end-of-life so we can live every day to its fullest, die comfortably, and give our families immense peace about our death?

Many people, at some point in their life, have a fear of dying. I am not an expert in this area, and many books have been written on this topic, but I will discuss a few practical things I have seen in my practice that make people afraid of dying. And I can offer tips from many of my patients who have died a peaceful, comfortable death.

1 "I Am Not Ready to Die – I Haven't Finished My Life's Work"

This is most true for younger people, who still have much to contribute. When older people make this statement, it is often not that they haven't accomplished enough – it is that they haven't consolidated their legacy to feel proud of themselves and grateful for a life well lived. Many people have accomplished a lot, but now they are older and feel less valuable to the world. This brings a sense of unease and reduced self-esteem that can lead to anxiety and fear of dying.

Much of what we discuss in this book will help bring meaning to later years. But it is also important to be able to look back on your life and identify the things of which you can be really proud: raising wonderful children, starting a business, making scientific discoveries or beautiful art, having a long happy relationship, providing care to a beloved family member. There comes a point for everyone when most accomplishments are behind us, and few accomplishments, if any, are before us. We have to be OK with this. I recommend sitting down with family and friends, and maybe even recording the conversations, to tell your life's story and let them help you appreciate your accomplishments. You will begin to understand the legacy you are leaving, and will be better able to reconcile with your death. As Wendy recommended in an earlier chapter, writing an ethical will can be a wonderful way to accomplish this milestone.

2 "I Am Afraid Death Will Be Painful and Very Uncomfortable"

This is an absolutely reasonable fear, and, unfortunately, some people do die with pain, shortness of breath, and other symptoms that make their death uncomfortable. But most people who plan well (as Mary did, despite her chronic and sometimes severe pain from her heart) do not have to die in pain. Their healthcare team can get hospice involved early enough to be able to provide superb symptom management. They can teach the family how to administer comfort medications, such as morphine for shortness of breath or lorazepam for end-of-life anxiety, to ensure a peaceful death. I recommend being very clear about your wishes by completing advance directives and a POLST form, as Mary did, to ensure that your family knows how to keep you comfortable. There are some great web-based tools to assist you in making future plans – Prepare for Your Care (https://prepareforyourcare .org/welcome) helps you work with your medical team to document your wishes and ensure that others know them. Another of my favorite resources is The Conversation Project (https://thecon versationproject.org) which walks you through many detailed questions to help you understand what your own wishes are and then help your family understand them too.

3 "I Am Afraid I Will Have a Long, Slow Death with Lots of Disability and Create a Heavy Burden for My Family"

Again, a very reasonable fear. None of us wants to live for a long time very disabled and reliant on a high level of care from family. This fear should be approached from a young age by doing all the things discussed in Wendy's chapters to ensure that you have adequate finances to help cover your care needs. So many of my patients have limited resources throughout life and nothing extra to set aside – but if you have the ability to live more frugally and set aside enough to be comfortable as you age, you can rest assured that you will not be a burden. If that isn't possible, I encourage you to seek out resources before you become disabled, whether they be through Medicaid, Meals on Wheels, the Alzheimer Association, community groups like the Villages, or others. Your primary care provider may have a social worker in their clinic who can help you understand what resources are available before you need them. Many people never learn what resources are available to them, and rely on their family more than they need to, or die less comfortably because they haven't tapped into the available resources.

4 "I Just Don't Know What Dying Is Like"

True. This is something most of us experience only once. I recommend talking with family members and friends who are close to death. Spend time with them. You will bring them comfort by your presence and caring, and you will also be able to ask them questions to learn more about dying. So many of us are afraid to talk about dying. Don't be afraid. If you don't have anyone near you who is growing older and getting closer to death, volunteer with a local hospice agency to be a companion for people who are dying. The hospice team will train you how to use the best words to bring comfort. The hospice patient will be so grateful for your time, and you will learn so much about dying. Also read Mitch Albom's *Tuesdays with Morrie*, Atul Gawande's *Being Mortal*, Sherwin Nuland's *How We Die*.

Once you have taken the time and trouble to work through your fears of dying, you can really start planning for a good death. It seems entirely possible to me that Mary chose to die on Christmas, after a lovely caroling session with her entire family around her. I have had patients who had been lingering, and then died peacefully when a daughter visited from England, or a grandchild successfully graduated from college, or a great-grandchild was born. Medicine tells us we are not in control of when we die. But my patient experiences tell me otherwise – at least, for some people. The more you can think through what you think would be your best possible death, and then plan for it, the more likely it will happen. I had a patient who wanted tulips next to her bed, and a family member brought three bunches of tulips to fulfill that wish. Most people want to die in their sleep before they are even sick, but in reality this is rare.

Think through which family members or friends will be comforting at your death bed. Think about those who won't be comforting, and be sure they aren't there. Another delightful patient invited her grandchildren to join her as she was dying. A 13-year-old boy spent several hours holding her hand and telling her about his math class (it was his favorite). She had a beautiful smile on her face as she gradually stopped breathing. My guess is she didn't comprehend what he was saying, but his voice was exactly what she wanted to hear as she died. Hearing is our last sense that we lose as we die, so peaceful talking at your deathbed is a big plus.

What does dying look like? As someone approaches death, the following things are very common:

1   They will have decreased oral intake, and will no longer eat or drink much. This does not cause discomfort – it is normal and they will not feel hungry or thirsty. This is hard for families to watch – they feel that, if their family member would only eat and drink, everything would be better! But it is a natural part of dying, and forcing a dying person to eat and drink is uncomfortable and anxiety-provoking. Families can provide sips of water, ice chips, or mouth swabs to reduce the sensation of dry mouth once eating and drinking stops.

2   Breathing changes. Breaths become shallow and frequent. A Cheyne–Stokes pattern of breathing (gradually increasing rate and depth of breaths, then gradually decreasing rate and depth breaths, then a period with no breaths at all) is very common. Nothing needs to be done for this; it is not uncomfortable.

3   Oral secretions build up. As swallowing becomes challenging, saliva can build up and cause "rattling" breaths. Hospice team members can provide medications to help this.

4   Confusion worsens. Most people become delirious (sometimes very somnolent, sometimes alert and maybe agitated) at the end of life. They will often talk about "going home," "joining my husband," or other death references. The hospice team can assist with medications – but medications are only needed if these symptoms seem to be causing distress.

5   There is diminished perfusion, causing low blood pressure, rapid heart rate, feeling cold, turning blue, and having mottled skin. These are all signs that death is approaching and are completely normal.

Most people spend hours to a few days in the active phase of dying. Hospice team members are excellent at helping families understand exactly how long to expect their family member to live once they start actively dying. They can show family members how to dose medications to keep their loved one comfortable, and can offer therapies like music, pets, and maybe acupuncture to make dying more comfortable. They can provide spiritual care if desired. And they can help surviving family members work through their grief – more about that in Chapter 30.

I have to tell one more story. I had a 95-year-old patient with advanced dementia who hadn't spoken in about 6 months. He had a loving nephew with whom he lived, and who ensured that he was comfortable, helped him get out for walks, and hired caregivers when his needs became very high. One day, the nephew called me and said "He is repeatedly reciting the Lord's Prayer." This surprised me; I didn't remember this patient as a religious person. The nephew reassured me that I wasn't remembering incorrectly. His uncle had only a third-grade education. The nephew had known him all his life and never known him to be religious in any way. And don't forget – he hadn't spoken a word in 6 months! The nephew reported that his uncle otherwise seemed to be doing fine. I hadn't seen him for a few months, but he was fine then. I told the nephew that I suspected his uncle was dying. I called hospice and asked them to go out and evaluate the patient because of his repetitive recitation of the Lord's Prayer! Luckily this was a hospice agency I worked with regularly, so they agreed to do it. Sure enough, the patient was repeatedly reciting the Lord's Prayer but was otherwise still up and moving a little, not eating but drinking some fluids. They admitted him to hospice. Within days, he developed Cheyne–Stokes breathing, low blood pressure, and agitation. Family members came from around the country to say good-bye. My patient died comfortably with family present – exactly three weeks after the nephew reported his reciting the Lord's Prayer. I will never forget that story.

I suspect most of us won't have the remarkable end-of-life experience that Susan's mother had, or that my 95-year-old patient had. Each death is unique. But if we work through our fears, plan as best we can, and talk with our primary care provider about getting hospice in a timely way, we can die comfortably, with a good ending, and leave our family feeling peaceful about our death.

There are only two things, two assets we have that matter in this life. They are love and time. It is how you spend this time, and how you spend your love, that tells you who you are.

Governor Barbara Roberts,
age 85

29 ONLY TWO THINGS

Marcy Cottrell Houle

It feels like an oxymoron. This sunny room, filled with pictures, wood carvings, potted plants, and copious books seems an unlikely place to bring up the subject of grief. Even more contradictory, the couple sitting in comfortable living-room chairs across from me exude such cheerfulness it seems capable of banishing any mention of sadness.

But this is why I'm here, to ask them some difficult questions. I know that grief is a multifaceted experience; dealing with it is as varied as the people going through it. Both these people have suffered the heartbreaking loss of a beloved spouse. Both are quick to say grieving is the hardest work a person can do, and it takes time, time, time. Yet they also profess that there is recovery, and, for Barbara Roberts and Don Nelson, something completely unexpected – falling in love again, at 80 and 88.

"There is no right or wrong way to grieve," says Barbara. "There is just your way."

I am interested in learning their ways, as the likelihood of losing a spouse or someone you deeply love is something many will face, especially on the journey of aging. I had gone through grief losing my beloved mother and father. It took a long time to get through the fog, the numbness.

"Part of grief will stay with you forever. I'm not sure you can ever fully mend when someone you love has died," Barbara says. "I have learned, though, that you can be happy again. When thinking about them, you can smile before you cry. You can laugh once more, enjoy music and flowers, and find reasons to begin again. But there is no time limit for healing. It can't be rushed. It's a long climb back, after losing someone you love."

Barbara's climb began four years before her husband died, with his diagnosis of advanced prostate cancer, which eventually took his life. Her grief had an added complexity most of us don't have to deal with. She and her husband Frank were both prominent public figures.

Barbara Roberts is a former governor of Oregon – the first woman governor ever elected in the state. At the time she served, from 1991 to 1995, she was 1 of only 10 women ever elected to that position in the United States. Scaffolding Barbara's achievements was the constant encouragement of her husband, Senator Frank Roberts, a two-time Oregon state legislator and Oregon state senator.

For 20 years, Barbara and Frank shared a very happy marriage. He remained in the State Senate for five terms. She was elected twice to the Oregon House of Representatives and served two terms as Oregon Secretary of State before becoming governor in 1991. Both husband and wife held remarkable records of progressive politics – advocating for the environment, civil rights, rights for disabled children, human rights, and higher education. Frank was known as the "conscience of the Senate." Barbara, highly thought of and well loved then and now, successfully passed 800 bills by the end of her term as governor.

In her third year as Oregon's governor, however, Barbara faced the greatest test she had ever encountered, one that up-ended her life: Frank's death.

"On October 31, 1993, the love of my life died. After months of knowing and preparing and dreading, the husband I loved was gone."

"How did you handle it?" I ask.

"I had my family, and I had work I had to do. It was always worse at night, when I would come home to the empty governor's mansion. All I could do was weep. At first, I needed private time to grieve alone. I felt I was living in a fog. I found it difficult to concentrate. It took a long time for joy to return."

The use of the word 'joy' in this context comes back again to strike me. I remember another conversation – with Rabbi Josh Stampfer. He spoke of his beloved wife, Goldie, who died several years ago. They had been married for 66 years. He talked about her, and of her death, and why he was not afraid of his own death. I then posited a difficult question to him: "Rabbi, there are a lot of people who, as they get older and lose those they love, become afraid to meet new people, fearing that they too will die and they will just have loved and lost again. And they fear their own death. How do you reconcile that?"

I remember the old rabbi's eyes were very kind as he replied.

"I will answer from my own case. What you say is true. But what is also true is that I'm perfectly willing to die tomorrow without any regrets. Every day really is wonderful for me. I realize that time is very finite. The only thing we can do is to make it as full as possible. That's where I find my joy."

"But what if you lose someone you deeply love?" I pressed on, thinking of Goldie.

Josh nodded. "When someone you deeply love dies? You absorb it. Do you know what the word absorb means? It means taking it into yourself. You'll never lose your memories. They are a part of you. What you have lost is the physical presence.

"I have found that memories can sometimes be even more fulfilling than the actual presence," said Josh. "When I go to sleep at night, I reach out my hand. I think I am holding Goldie's hand. And it feels good."

I observe Barbara reaching over to say something to Don, lay her hand lightly on his, then sit back again. She turns toward me.

"You never forget the one you love who has died. Don and I talk about our late spouses. They're okay topics. In fact," she says, "we can joke about them."

"Joke about them?"

"For example, Leslie did not swim," Barbara begins.

"Leslie was my wife," Don interjects. "We were married for 54 years before she died several years ago."

"And I don't swim," Barbara continues. "Leslie hated the dentist, and I hate the dentist. We both love to play the slot machines."

"If the two of them had met – " Don starts.

"We would have been best friends," says Barbara. "I'm sure of it!"

"The other thing they have in common?" Don says; "Leslie made me laugh and she," pointing at Barbara, "makes me laugh."

At that, she does laugh. "We feel so fortunate to feel the joy that we feel," Barbara concurs. "But of course, it took a long time." She becomes thoughtful. "Every person who goes through suffering is different, I believe. Eventually I could recall memories of Frank without feeling stabs of pain. You come through the haze and relentless seas of grief. My first glimpses of recovery happened two years after Frank died. I surprised myself. I found I could actually laugh again, laugh out loud."

I reflect how long it took me to laugh again after my mother died. I actually can remember the exact moment when the fog lifted. It helped to talk about it with John. And I attended a hospice grief support group. They provided books, had questions for us to consider, and helped me understand the cycles better.

"Rituals can help, or at least they helped me," Barbara continues. "I made a photo album of 50 precious pictures of Frank and special times we spent together. I would look at it every evening. For two years I kept it on the table by my bed. I also collected some of his personal belongings – like his wallet and glasses – and displayed them around the house where I could see them. Just knowing they were there made him feel closer."

"What did you do, Don?" I ask. "Did you have rituals?"

Thinking for a moment, Don shakes his head. "Not rituals, per se. For me, I think it helped to stay busy. Or perhaps being busy was just an escape. After Leslie died, I repainted rooms, took wallpaper down, just kept busy doing stuff. In time, I had a couple of blind dates. They were disasters! So I gave up the thought. In time, loneliness really manifests. But I did something that really helped."

"What was that?"

"I think becoming isolated is the case for lots of widows and widowers," he says. "Or maybe anybody who suffers a loss. When Leslie was in the hospital for the last time, she got many wonderful cards that meant a lot. After she died, I got many more wonderful cards. But before long those cards stop coming. Everyone moves on. People quit calling. I think it's that people don't know if they are supposed to call, or if they do call, what to say."

"What did you do that helped?" I asked, curious.

"I came up with a plan."

"Really, quite brilliant," declares Barbara, smiling.

"I started calling my friends, beginning with my oldest friends and working backwards. When they answered, they'd invariably ask how I was doing. 'Fine,' I'd say. But then I'd say, 'Would you do me a favor?' Being friends, of course they'd say yes. So I'd deliver the punchline: 'Will you invite me to dinner?'"

"You're audacious!" laughs Barbara.

"I'd go! And after that meal, I'd work down the list. I'd call the next family and the next family. Eventually, I didn't have to ask myself over for dinner anymore. It just became natural ... doing things with friends."

"I think the reason it worked so well," Barbara offers, "is that many times people don't know how to reach out to you once your spouse has died."

"Well, it did work very well," Don agrees. "Frankly, they all sounded relieved."

Don's blue eyes are twinkling and the energy between these two fills the room with warmth. Still, I know it takes more than rituals and dinners with friends to find healing. Also, I am curious why such a much-loved governor as Barbara didn't run for a second term. Most Oregonians thought she would and it would have been an easy race for her to win.

"Campaigning is never easy," Barbara acknowledges when I bring up the question. "One needs tremendous energy and enthusiasm to take on such a demand. I was still grieving Frank's death. I loved Oregon, and cared deeply about my work as governor. I could not envision campaigning, fundraising, television spots, and polling numbers so soon after he died. While he was ill, Frank had encouraged me to run again, but I made the choice to withdraw from my re-election race. At a different time, the choice would have been different. But at the time, I knew it was the right decision."

"What did you do?"

"After my term was up, I went to Harvard."

Barbara explains she accepted a position at Harvard University, teaching and running leadership programs at the

Kennedy School of Government. While she enjoyed it, she longed for Oregon. After five years she returned home, taking a job as Associate Director of Leadership Development at the Hatfield School of Government at Portland State University.

The work of healing was not over yet, however. What she learned, she said, was the importance of 'listening.'

"Grief waits its turn and will not go away until it has been heard. It's essential, I believe, to give ourselves permission to grieve in our own time and in our own way."

Part of that way, for Barbara, was to write a book. Nine years after her term as governor, she published a highly acclaimed volume about her mourning experiences, *Death without Denial: Grief without Apology*. She discovered she loved the writing process. Plus, it allowed for more public speaking and opportunities to reach out to others.

"I discovered that we all carry deep, hidden grief somewhere in our hearts," she says. "Sharing our tears brings people together."

"Is that when you met Don?" I ask.

"Heavens no. I had to write another whole book first."

"*Up the Capitol Steps*," breaks in Don. "Love that book. If it weren't for that book, I doubt I would be sitting here now!"

"That and your great line," adds Barbara.

"It was a great line, wasn't it? And it worked!"

Don leans forward to tell the story. "Several years after Leslie died, I read in the local newspaper that Governor Barbara Roberts was coming to King City, where I lived, to do a book reading. I had met Barbara 30 years before, but knew she wouldn't remember me. Her husband, Frank, the state senator, had also chaired the communications department at Portland State. He helped pass a bill to license speech pathologists. I'm a speech pathologist. I worked for years at Oregon Health and Science University, and at the time the bill was being lobbied I was President of the Speech and Hearing Association.

"I went to the signing," he continues, with a sheepish grin, "and hung around while she was autographing books. I waited for the perfect moment, when she was packing things up. I drummed up all my courage to say, 'Can I carry your books for you?'"

"They were heavy! So I let him."

Don's house, he explains, was only a block from her car. He asked if she would like to sit on his deck and have a cold beer.

"I can't believe I got that bold!" he says.

"I can't believe I said yes!" Barbara laughs.

"We sat and talked for an hour. When she got ready to go, I asked her one more question. 'What would happen if I called you for lunch?'"

Now Barbara is sitting forward on her chair too, smiling at him. "I told him, 'Why don't you call me for lunch and find out?' And I gave him my card! For a minute, I regretted it! Remember, I hadn't dated anyone in 20 years and this was a big step!"

They did have that lunch. And talked. Several days later, they went on a picnic. Then to a museum. They ate out in the park. They realized they both had similar interests and values, and both derived pleasures from simple things.

"I delight in the beauty of Oregon. Don does too. We find joy just standing and looking up at a big, gorgeous cedar tree. We love seeing the sparkling water of the Willamette River near our home. We don't need a tropical island with a crew to cook our dinner. That's phony. We would much prefer walking together on a nice summer evening, appreciating Mt. Hood, feeding our souls – on Oregon."

Don and Barbara will be celebrating their eighth anniversary in two months; they are already planning for that day. The love they share does not erase the grief they both endured, nor does it diminish the years of the work of healing. As I can see, looking at them, the grief has been incorporated into the rich fabric of their lives, magnifying their sense of gratitude for living.

Sitting on a shelf beside Barbara is an exquisite wood carving of a hawk. Barbara catches me admiring it.

"It is beautiful, isn't it? The hawk was Frank's favorite bird. The carving always reminds me of him. When he knew he was dying, he told me there are only two things, two assets we have that matter in this life. They are love and time. It is how you spend this time, and how you spend your love, that tells you who you are."

30 GRIEF AND LOSS

Normal Parts of Aging. Not to Be Missed

Elizabeth Eckstrom, MD, MPH, MACP

I bet every one of us who had a pet as a child remembers when they died. We remember the grief we felt, and the belief that we could never love a pet – or maybe anything or anyone – again. But with time, we bounced back, and finally were able to get the new puppy that allowed us to be fully joyful and in love again. Death is a normal part of life. Grief is a normal part of life. Without grief, we have not loved deeply. Consider it a privilege to grieve – it means you have loved well.

But it is important to understand grief so that you can make your way through it and recognize red flags for when you should seek help. I am sure everyone has heard of the "stages of grief" – shock/denial, anger, bargaining, depression, acceptance. These are not linear and one can experience any of these symptoms at any time in the grieving process – from the date of a diagnosis of a life-limiting disease to many years after the death of a loved one. Rather, I am going to ask and then hopefully answer some questions about grief that may help guide you through it, and even help you understand better what to expect if it hasn't affected you yet.

1 **What is normal grief?**

I love the quote from Barbara Roberts: "There is no right or wrong way to grieve . . . just your way." My patients and medical textbooks describe many symptoms of grief. Physical symptoms can include crying, fatigue, headache, abdominal pain, sleep disturbance (too much or too little), eating disturbance (too much or too little), pain, unhealthy behaviors like drinking too much, forgetfulness, and many others. When someone you love has died, it is okay to cry 100 times a day! And if you don't cry at all right away, that's okay too. Your body is grieving in different ways, and you may cry eventually. I have had patients feel guilty that they weren't crying more. There is no reason to feel guilty! Some people want to be alone after a loved one dies, and some people want to be with others to distract them from the loneliness. Either option is okay; the important thing is that it is *your* way. Many people are angry, frustrated, anxious, irritable, down, and feel guilty they didn't "do enough" for their loved one. All of this is normal. Another thing to remember: grief will hit you in *waves*. You may start to feel a little better, and then it will wash over you again. It is normal for this to last for months.

2   **When should I worry about my symptoms?**

All of these expressions of grief are totally normal, but I hope you can also "look over your own shoulder" enough to recognize when any of these symptoms are causing your health to deteriorate. I encourage everyone who has lost an important person in their life to see their primary care provider to tell them about it, and discuss the symptoms they are experiencing, even if they are normal and don't require intervention. Your provider will offer words of solace and wisdom that will help you through this time. But they will also help recognize when something needs to be done. You may feel down and anxious, have difficulty sleeping and eating. Your provider can help identify if these are leading to decline in your health. If you are gaining or losing weight, not exercising regularly, losing sleep, anxious enough that it is impairing your daily function, or having other symptoms – while all normal – it still may be useful to take an antidepressant or anti-anxiety medication for a few months.

Medications such as sertraline (Zoloft® in the US, Lustral® in the UK) and escitalopram (Lexapro® in the US, Cipralex® in the UK) are excellent antidepressant/anti-anxiety agents that can also help energy and concentration. Mirtazapine is another great antidepressant/anti-anxiety agent that can help improve sleep and appetite. Melatonin, a natural product that can help "reset your clock" and improve your sleep, might be needed to get through the tough parts of the grieving process. These medications are generally safe for older people.

Don't feel like you should "tough it out" – that will not help you be your best self as you come out the other end!

3 **How long will grief last?**

Medical professionals are trained to think that normal grief lasts about 3–12 months. But it clearly can last far longer. Barbara Roberts described a much longer, but still normal, grieving process. I agree with her that we can continue to feel grief even after we have completely recovered from the loss. It can simply be a reminder of the wonderful person who was close to us for a very long time! Keep mementos handy – photos, personal items, whatever reminds you of the joy you shared – to bring you solace when your grief strikes again.

4 **How can I prepare for the loss of someone with a life-limiting illness?**

This is a really tough question. Many older people are faced with a terrible diagnosis like late-stage cancer, and their spouse or partner has to be the caregiver and provide comfort as well as assistance. But all the while, that partner is also realizing that the afflicted care partner will have health decline so they are not the person they were before. They comprehend the painful reality that they will be alone once their partner dies.

Even worse, many partners are faced with a loved one's new diagnosis of dementia. This means they may begin to suffer the loss of their partner's cognition long before that person actually dies. Grief in dementia starts years before death and often extends years after death.

In Chapter 24, I write about "caring for the caregiver." This is essential to preparing for the loss of a loved one. So many times, a caregiver actually dies before the loved one with a life-limiting diagnosis because they have worked so tirelessly to provide comfort that they have neglected their own needs.

I reiterate, please do something every day to stay healthy! And, I honestly advise, let yourself *think* about what life will be like after your loved one dies. You are going to need a support team. If you are sequestering yourself to care on your own for your loved one, you won't have that support team once your loved one is gone. Foster your team *now*. It is perfectly fine to dream about a trip you will make, a cozy small apartment instead of a big house, family time you will spend with grandchildren – all of the things that will help you recover from the loss of your life partner.

Remember, most importantly, don't go through your grief alone. Even if it feels better to isolate most of the time, be sure you have someone with whom to talk. If your partner was on hospice before they died, the hospice team can provide a support group and other resources. Even if your partner wasn't on hospice, you can ask your provider for a hospice referral to tap into these resources. And follow your own heart on how to get through grief. I love Don's strategy of inviting himself to dinner at all of his friends' houses – oldest ones first! And follow Barbara and Don's lead to let yourself love again.

The pain of loss may be terrible, but "'Tis better to have loved and lost than never to have loved at all" (Alfred Lord Tennyson). Your loved one will be in your heart and mind for the rest of your life.

It is worth it.

Everyone must understand their obligation to the next
generation. Especially as we grow older.

David Barrios,
age 77

31 LIVING TO MAKE A DIFFERENCE

Marcy Cottrell Houle

The freshness of the springtime meadow is enhanced by the singing of yellow warblers coming from the bigleaf maple trees. It seems the perfect place to talk to David Barrios, park ranger for Forest Park, to ask him about something that continues to trouble me. At 77, David, an Indigenous elder in the urban Native community of Portland, Oregon, has told me that the Indigenous perspective on aging is different from what I am used to seeing in our current culture. And after what I went through with my parents, I am curious to see whether this might be yet another trailside marker on my map of the aging journey.

In years of caring for both my mother and father as they aged, I saw something that alarmed me. As they grew older and developed more health problems, they seemed to become, in our present-day society, increasingly un-noticed. Worse, when my wonderful father, a beloved physician and surgeon for most of his adult life, developed Alzheimer Disease, he not only became more and more invisible to the world, but someone to be avoided. I saw a terrible truth that, regardless of their years-long history of service and wisdom, when many people get old they are effectively pushed out of society as they are increasingly perceived as less useful. Worse, what they come to experience is something none of them ever wished for: feeling they are a burden to their family.

Sitting next to me on a park bench, David smiles. He looks official and youthful in his park ranger uniform – more than that, he appears entirely relaxed and comfortable with himself and the natural surroundings. "That is not the way it is for us," he says. "When I grew up, I learned quickly how very important it was culturally to be not only respectful of your elders but responsible for caring for them. We understand this is where our knowledge base comes from. Our grandparents teach us our values and what comes in life. I guess you could say my orientation on aging is the way of my ancestors – Indigenous people of northern Mexico and southwestern Texas, east of the Rio Grande. They were from Apacheria, the domain of the Apache people. My grandmother was Jumano Mescalero, a member of an Apache tribe that originally inhabited these southwestern lands before being driven out by Indian wars and the Mexican Revolution."

But David did not grow up in the southwest.

"Unfortunately, I was born in the City of Chicago. I say that in complete deference to what Chicagoans feel is their home," he continues. "But for me, without the natural world, it was like a lifeless zone. I grew up in an old neighborhood with houses built after the Great Chicago Fire in the 1870s. We had old buildings without central heating. Our neighborhoods were crowded, rough, and smelled of pig iron foundries. My people had come from the country, but I was a kid stuck in the city."

Chicago used to be a hub, David explains, for Indigenous resettlement, as part of the government's policy of indoctrinating Native people to blend into society. It was there that he grew up with his grandparents.

"I asked my grandmothers lots of questions. Both were born in the 1880s. When they were children, it was the tail-end of the Apache Wars. Geronimo was still active and was not captured until 1886. People rode horses and moved around in wagons, and Indian people were still at war with governments in Mexico and the United States. The knowledge that my grandmothers brought to me was knowledge you can't get anywhere else.

"In Native communities, elders are held in very high esteem. I loved listening to their stories. They were rancho people, rural people, farmers. Everything they told me just added to my thirst to be in the natural world."

David left Chicago in his late teens, moving to Oregon with a close friend. After college, he went into police work in Portland, Oregon, and the Columbia River Gorge. He later became a tribal officer and did training with other tribal officers on reservations all across the country. While many of the tribes he visited had different traditions, common amongst them all, David says, was the importance of elders.

"You check up on the elders. You make sure they have food and wood for the winter. As a Native person, you know that elders are the people who have the experience," he shares. "They know the prayers. The *old* prayers. They know the language. They know the course of history that your tribe has been through, and the trials and tribulations they experienced. They also have the keys to all the ceremonies and the way things are done. They are our teachers. That's why we rely on our elders."

In 2006, David at last began doing the work he had always wanted to do – as a park ranger. For the last 16 years, he has helped families and children understand the riches and gifts in our parks, and how to care for these in a loving way. As he speaks, I notice what seems to be a small basket that he is wearing on a string around his neck. He catches my gaze.

"I wear this little basket to remind me of my growing up. Baskets are very important in understanding our Native values. When I was born, I was put in a basket and brought home. That basket symbolized that I was a valuable person, a cherished new entry into the family. As I grew a little older, as a toddler, I was put in a bigger basket. Everything my grandmothers and my mother and my elders valued were always in baskets. Their special medicines. Their jewelry. Food too, of course, went into baskets. It is symbolic for us that baskets hold meaningful things, just like the birds build a basket in the tree to hold their young. Through baskets, you begin to understand the symbology in your life right away. They remind you of what you need to remember."

I like that ... what you need to remember. What was I forgetting?

David looks at the meadow stretching out before us – healthy, green grass dotted with thousands of tiny white daisies. "Values are vital to carry you through life," he says. "You learn very quickly that elders are part of your life because they teach you what you need to know. Elders are the architects of the culture. They instill the traditions of your people. How to be respectful;

what is prohibited in your life; who came before you. To Native peoples, both young people and elders are indispensable."

"I wish we all felt that way," I say, reflecting that too often, in today's culture, it is the very young and very old who are most marginalized.

"We live in a difficult time," David agrees. "Today, the whole way we think is so different. Now we have the great distractions of technology – distractions that take us away from what our generations before gave to us. They cut off that flow of knowledge that came from elders and cannot be substituted by technology. With so much to distract us, it's hard for people to sit still for that kind of information. People don't go to their elders. They go to their phones when they want to think."

He stops to listen to the sounds of birds coming from around us, then looks at me. His face is kind.

"I am grateful. In Native communities, elders and young people are held in high esteem. Young people are the purpose for it all. That's why elders have an obligation. An obligation to stay with it, which means you don't just retire and go and play golf, and disappear. You have to stay with it, and help that next generation get through. Everyone must understand their obligation to the next generation, especially as we grow older. If we do not safeguard our earth for the next generation, we can lose so much very quickly. Native and non-native communities can learn from each other through the commonality of our need of the earth. We all need some soil under our feet to understand what our gifts are."

A friendly rufous-sided towhee catches our eyes. Working industriously, it is scratching the duff and needles searching for insects below a giant, old Douglas fir tree. The jaunty small black and red bird makes both of us smile.

"My work as a ranger is to help people form a positive relationship with parks," he says. "We invite people to enjoy nature in a medicinal way – which is so important in times like we are living through. It is spiritual medicine. When you are in nature, you are seeing life that is complex, but also very nurturing and healing and welcoming. When we walk in nature, we do a little dreaming, and wondering, and hoping. That's very much Native thinking."

I know David works with adults and children, helping them appreciate the Forest Park he loves. It is clear to me that, at nearly 80 years old, he is improving the quality of life in Portland. He has found meaning in his older years that many might envy.

"Our responsibility as elders only gets more vital as we grow older," he says, helping me to understand. "Many things don't have a voice. The natural world does not have a voice that can be interpreted by most people. Therefore, we have an obligation as elders to speak for the earth. It becomes increasingly important to inspire young people to care for the earth . . . to help them observe, to see and touch and smell and be in the natural world – to learn first-hand what is there. The more they know, the more they'll care. And the more wonder they'll have. They will have an understanding of the relationship they have to other things. The trees, the birds. Nature is our relative.

"You ask me what Native peoples think about aging," says David, thoughtfully. "We look at life in a circular way. Time is not linear. But I had a dream the other night that might help you think about your own journey into aging. Dreams are significant to Native people, and my dream made me think about the end of life, and the beginning of life."

He pauses, and I wonder what it might feel like to go through life thinking life is a circle, and not a line, especially as we grow old.

"When we are born, we believe that the Creator gives us the gift of youth," David continues. "We use that gift from infancy into adulthood. As we move through life, there are exchanges. When young people come together with old people, it is a blending of ages. Young people get the benefit of the age and wisdom of the older person, and the kindness and ways old people experience love and family. Old people experience a rejuvenation with the exposure to young people. Meaning is found in understanding our connections with others.

"But my dream told me something more," he adds. "Whereas the Creator gives you youth, as you grow older, youth is the gift you give *yourself*. As you age, you can give yourself the gift of life in the *narrative* you tell yourself. You have the power to say the self-motivating words, 'I still have that youth inside. I will take that gift, given to me by my Creator, and use it again.'

"It is too easy to convince ourselves that we are too old to walk, too old to run, or to get on a bike, or take up ballroom dancing or even go parachuting! We tell ourselves things that limit our thinking about what we can do. What is happening is that we haven't stopped to give ourselves that gift of youth that was given to us at our birth.

"What my dream told me is that you *always* have the gift of youth inside you. But it's up to you to rekindle it and to bring it back. It will give you the energy to renew your commitment to helping others. You are mustering up those youthful values, and recalling the experiences you remember that were solid and good. It is our duty as elders to live, not just for ourselves, but for the generations of young people coming after us and for the earth."

For a moment we sit in silence. Reflecting on his words, I begin to see the pivotal role elders could play in determining our future. Instead of vanishing from society, feeling outdated and of decreasing value, older people need to understand their worth.

We need to recognize what is the true gift of aging.

For the first time in human history, seniors are living longer than ever before. We have been given additional years to try to help our hurting world, to try to make a difference in our fragmented communities, and to work to benefit the lives of those coming after us.

As David says, that's just what elders are here to do.

Another trail marker has been hewn for me, a new direction-finder on my map:

Make that time count.

Each morning I wake up, I am grateful, you know, because I know there are spirits among us who did not wake up this morning. As long as I wake up, I've got another shot. I've got another turn at bat. I've got another chance to hit the ball out of the ballpark.

Karen Wells,
age 70

32 THE GREAT LEVELER

Marcy Cottrell Houle

Aging is the great leveler. If we live long enough, we all grow old. And the finish line is the same for all of us. But, of course, as I've learned, the path we take toward the end makes a big difference to our state of health, well-being, safety, and happiness as we pass through this part of our journey. Some routes are clearer than others. Some have high obstacles.

It is in these final laps where aging's great divergences are revealed. Standing at this crossroads, looking both ahead and behind me, I begin to understand Elizabeth's deep belief – and worry – that our trek needs to be done as a community. We cannot leave our friends and neighbors behind.

"In the focus on healthy aging, African Americans have always been at a disadvantage. We've been left out," says Karen Wells, as we sit around her dining-room table on a cool early February afternoon. "We grow old, too, but often without the benefits of having good healthcare. That's why my mission, if you'd call it that, is to grow the body of work as it pertains to communities of color."

I am here just for that reason: to learn more about PreSERVE – the coalition for African American Memory and Brain Health. The association is composed of community members and representatives from healthcare organizations and non-profits in Portland, Oregon. Its aim is to empower older African Americans to maintain and improve brain health through a healthy lifestyle. Karen, almost 70, has been an active member since learning about the association in 2012.

"We host monthly meetings where people can learn, socialize, and exercise, while focusing on the health issues that exist in many communities of color. We pay special attention to those problems that can impact brain health – high blood pressure, diabetes, and dementia. I've been involved in workshops and conferences since PreSERVE first appeared on my radar," says Karen.

Karen, who was an early childhood development educator, currently writes for the neighborhood newspaper, participates in her local American Association of Retired Persons (AARP) chapter, and is deeply involved in the monthly meetings PreSERVE puts on for the community. As well, she helps plan for the larger-scale events PreSERVE has held over the past few years.

"Our local gatherings center on a wide range of topics that affect older people of color and aid them to learn helpful strategies. Sometimes we've had as many as four events a year. We've had meetings on Tips for Healthy Aging, How to Stay Steady on Your Feet, Get Out and Walk!, Stress and Mindfulness, the Joys and Sorrows of Caregiving, and we also put on a conference on Aging and Memory in the African American Community. We're involved with Oregon Health and Science University, advocating for recruiting young up-and-coming researchers who are people of color.

"None of this can come soon enough," she makes clear. "Sometimes I use an attorney's term for what many African Americans face health-wise as they age: 'Death by 1,000 cuts.' It starts at birth. It's not the one cut that will kill you, but it's the accumulative effect that will do a person in."

Affirming that long, treacherous trajectory, a recent study of 32 million births in the US reveals the disparities among them. Karen is correct. Poor health outcomes start at birth. Research shows that pregnant women exposed to high temperatures or air pollution are more likely to have children who are premature, underweight, or stillborn, and the effects hurt African American mothers and babies most.

Karen continues to explain about the early childhood classes she ran to warn parents about the dangers of lead exposure from older pipes in their homes. Many in her community have lead-infused pipes.

"Again, I would tell them it's not the one-time exposure that will harm your child but the accumulative exposure that will hurt them. Think of Flint, Michigan's public health crisis when its drinking water was found to be contaminated and exposed thousands of children to lead. I guess you'd say my whole life, I have wanted to make things better. Back in my 20s, I was going to save the world! I learned, however, the 'ism' sisters are tough to fight."

Reflecting momentarily, she counts them off on her fingers.

"Classism. Misogynism. Racism. Ageism. And, of course, over and above it all, there is white privilege. In time, I discovered I could not save the world from all the inequities. I had to come to terms with what things I wanted to commit my life-blood to. Right now, the major one I'm involved with is the inequality in healthcare, especially as it pertains to old people and communities of color. Of course, ageism exists in all communities."

Experts on aging confirm that. Joanne Lynn, MD, a geriatrician and Director of the Altarum Institute to Improve Elder Care, has spent her professional life trying to increase awareness of how our society ignores the needs of old people. She exhorts us all that we need to start paying attention *now*, because the outcomes for all baby boomers, no matter who you are, will over time become worse . . . much worse.

A century ago, Dr. Lynn says, most older Americans had multiple descendants. Many lived on a farm, and family members were available to provide necessary support. Today, however, family structure has changed dramatically. Families are smaller; they live farther apart; older caregivers have their own disabilities.

Add to that new population dynamics. The population of those over 80 will increase by nearly *80%* in the next 10 years! Research predicts that, between 2015 and 2050, the number of frail and disabled adults needing long-term supportive services will more than double. There simply aren't going to be enough younger people to care for their needs.

"Old age looks to become grim for most Americans," says Dr. Lynn. "There will be fewer family caregivers, a low supply of healthcare workers, inadequate personal savings, and declines in pension plans. Many older Americans who live with disabilities will not be able to pay for adequate housing, food, medicine, and personal care."

Karen nods her head in agreement at these frightening statistics.

"I know many families of color – black, brown, and Native – that are unable to pay for healthcare, and so fundamentally they receive none. In this sort of system, no one benefits."

"So what can we do?" I ask, overwhelmed with the task ahead.

"You try to do your best for your community. But I've learned the key is to pace yourself. Be selective in your confrontations. Because," she says with the smallest trace of a smile, "if you survive to the next moment, it means you'll get another chance."

She leans forward and puts her hands together on the table.

"The point is we must never give up. We need to help each other, to build up the human connection among us. To engage. It reminds me of a practice I saw growing up. People would sit out on their porch, and that was a good thing. Why? Because they're out of their house, getting fresh air and they can engage with their community as they walk by.

"We are social creatures. If we get cut off from people, which is easy to do when you're old and compromised, it can lead you into a downward spiral to depression and anxiety. Add to that your senses often begin to deteriorate. You may lose vision and hearing, even smell and taste. But having someone else in a room with you tells you, you aren't alone. It is a *ministry of presence*. As long as you are present in the moment, you have the opportunity to give."

I am inspired by Karen's caring and strength while thinking about the many biases, discrimination, and unfairness suffered by people we marginalize in our communities and our country. And, as I learn from talking with Dr. Lynn, it's only going to become more injurious as we grow old as a population, unless policies change. In the papers she writes, Dr. Lynn is clear on this scenario, calling for "the fierce urgency of now" – the phrase the Reverend Martin Luther King, Jr., used in his "I Have a Dream" speech. Dr. Lynn insists that everyone who serves older adults has an obligation and an opportunity to act *now*. The suffering that is in store for us *can* be averted. If we fail, though, as Dr. Lynn reminds us, old age will be uncertain for all and enkindle misery for countless people. We can do better. We must.

"Do you like to garden?" Karen asks me, startling me out of my reverie.

"Gardening? Um, sure."

"When you asked me 'Where do I find my strength and joy?' I'd say it all goes back to gardening," Karen says. "Weeding in particular. Weeding is one of those activities that require full body engagement. It addresses fine and gross motor skills as well as balance and cognition. When you feel you don't have agency or control over a particular situation, weeding is wonderful because you go out there and you can actually pull something out and have an end result that's positive and productive." She smiles. "And it's always available to you, always going to be there. You're never done."

Suddenly the room feels brighter. And for the first time since coming to her home, I notice all the plants around her house, and beds of early spring flowers and shrubs burgeoning outside every window.

"I am a gardener," she continues, briskly. "I may not be as bouncy as I was, it's harder getting down to the ground and standing back up, but that's okay. I've learned to pace myself. I garden plants, people, and projects. I grow them, they prosper, they go through their phases. Those things are important to me. I don't require grandiose things to be happy. I learned early that the simple pleasures in life are the most reliable. Because the big ones? They are intermittent. Sometimes the biggest ones are the most disappointing, because, after the ramping up, the whole drama, it's like, 'Is this all it is?'

"Indeed, it's the little things, the small triumphs, and the natural world that drive me. They provide an anchor and a foundation."

That foundation is on my map, but Karen has given me another clue to direction-finding. On this journey we all partake in, our skin tones might look different, we may have different religious beliefs, come from different native cultures, or have totally unrelated backgrounds, but we will only succeed on our path to healthy aging if we realize we are *all in it together*. We need to see ourselves as part of a greater whole – that we are connected as *one family*. We need to look out for one another. Working together from start to finish.

There is a long way to go.

"Each morning I wake up, I am grateful, you know, because I know there are spirits among us who did not wake up this morning," Karen says. "As long as I wake up, I've got another shot. I've got another turn at bat. I've got another chance to hit the ball out of the ballpark.

"And as long as I have another opportunity to make a difference, I will keep going."

When you get older you can see more deeply into things around you and get more satisfaction. The spiritual is coming at you, and it creates, if not a physical, but a mental and emotional adventure.

Neal Maine,
age 85

33 VIEW FROM THE MOUNTAIN

Marcy Cottrell Houle

The sound of the Pacific Ocean rhythmically pounds against the shore, the force of its crash buffered by the rich estuary below us, separating us from the sea. Dunes overgrown with beach grass slope down to the wet sand abounding with life. Sea gulls soar overhead; industrious sand-pipers poke along the beach.

This is the place that Neal Maine loves – the northern Oregon Coast – and for over a half-century has undertaken to save.

"There are messages coming to us from nature," says Neal, an 85-year-old retired science teacher and founder of North Coast Land Conservancy, "although we may not always recognize them – 95% of the world is unseeable to us; every piece of soil, every drop of water lets us know there is a whole world of nature churning away and generating phenomena that keep us alive."

He smiles, adding warmth to an already sunny morning in June. Neal has lived his entire life by the sea. He grew up near it, went to college, and, enamored with the seashore's teeming life, settled down to teach biology at the local high school, exposing hundreds of kids to the wonders of the ocean and its adjoining streams, wetlands, forests, and rugged mountains hugging the dunes. Driven by an intense appreciation of the natural beauty of the coast, Neal helped form one of the first land trusts in Oregon. Today, after five decades, Neal remains involved. The North Coast Land Conservancy has saved thousands of acres of native landscape from development, and is on the verge of creating a Rainforest Reserve unlike any other park in the nation.

But I am not here today to talk about Neal's accomplishments. Always humble, I know he would deflect attention away from himself anyway. A wheeling osprey circles above us, on the lookout for a fish. Neal picks up the binoculars from his lap to watch the beautiful raptor. I pick up mine too, but can't help first pinning my gaze on Neal's face. It's a kind, welcoming face, sculpted by sea wind, like that of an old ship's captain who has weathered storms only to love the sea all the more.

We sit on twin benches on the top of the dune. We have a splendid view of the beach, unpeopled and vast, extending for miles both north and south.

Today I want to know more about the *Art of Seeing* – Neal's newest venture, using photography to showcase the richness of the coastal landscape.

Neal places the binoculars back around his neck. "Look at your feet, Marcy."

Quickly, I glance down wondering what I might have stepped in. But it has nothing to do with my shoes. Leaning over, he points to a cheerful dandelion, pushing up through the grass. "That dandelion, if you knew everything it took for it to be a dandelion, would become the most amazing thing you could possibly see!" says Neal. "Taking time to regard that jolly flower, or a red flowering currant unfolding, or listening to a Pacific wren singing its heart out from the undergrowth, provides joy that can touch us at any age.

"At the end of some days when I have been outside, I can hardly believe I could have had a day like this one," Neal declares, with all the enthusiasm of a young boy. "Although I may not be able to walk as far, or bend down as long, or cross streams as easily as I once did, anytime I can see a beaver or great blue heron provides as much excitement as anything I can imagine. I would say life close to nature gets even better when you get older."

I find that statement fascinating. Neal has always appreciated nature and being outdoors, as do I, but it gets better as you get older? How?

"There are several reasons," says Neal. He points to a pair of Caspian terns flying like boomerangs, soaring back and forth over the beach. "I love watching the terns fly. I have watched them for many years. What is different now over time is that they have a context attached to them. When I see a tern, I think of where they nest, their young, their flight patterns and migration. What has changed is that I have developed *inventory*.

"When you're young, you're so busy talking that you don't spend much time listening. But as you mature, you can learn to stand on top of all that talking, and become a listener. You have a context now for all that talk; what you hear is being added to a structure that's in place. And as you move through life that inventory piles up.

"When you hear talk, there is more reference for it now, more meaning and evaluation. And this is not merely talk in words. Rather, it is messages that are coming at you. Messages from people and from nature. You can look and see and listen to what the estuaries and trees are saying and the landscape of nature."

I like the idea of added inventory and ask him to explain further.

"It is simple really. It's adding to the storehouse of knowledge you already have, which then becomes a new and richer base of experience," Neal says.

"But what about the art of seeing? What do you mean by that?"

"Thoreau spoke of it," Neal replies. "He said, 'It's not what you're looking at that matters, it's what you're *seeing*.' As I've grown older, I've learned if you are paying attention, the quality of your life goes up. Way up!

"When you work to develop the art of seeing, your world keeps getting bigger and bigger. That's what I hope to share in my pictures. It's helping people discover beauty where many don't think to look. I've found that a secret to getting older. When you slow down, you can find an exciting, beautiful world easy to miss when you're so busy racing your pace. Take for example, a beach walk," he says, waving his arm at the wide expanse of open sand before us. "When I was younger, my walks used to be from Point A to Point B. I just wanted to get there! Now my beach walks are A, B, C, D, and E. I am checking it all out along the way! I've moved from looking to seeing. And my whole world expands."

The black and white osprey, a master of flight and dive, swoops down and catches a salmon. For a moment we observe, unspeaking. Then Neal leans over to pick up a piece of driftwood from a pile next to us and lays it in my hand.

"My hope is, from my art, people can become responsive to the bigger pictures all around them. Look closely at that rotted piece of wood," he says. "There is a message in it. That remnant driftwood is different from any other piece on the entire beach. It has its own pattern, its own writing. It came from a tree; and no two trees are the same. That piece of driftwood is the message left by the tree."

Neal laughs again. "Yes, your pace gets slower; the name of that bird might not slip off your tongue as it once did. It may not be a Caspian tern after all but an Arctic tern. No matter. We are going for the beauty. When you get older you can see more deeply into things around you and get more satisfaction. The spiritual is coming at you, and it creates, if not a physical, but a mental and emotional adventure."

We pause to observe a bald eagle in pursuit of the osprey and its prize. For a moment I am reminded of special times I shared with my father, who also had a deep attachment to nature. We spent years walking and running and hiking together as a family. When he developed Alzheimer Disease, and finally had to go to a memory care center, his time outdoors was greatly reduced. But whenever I could take him outdoors, his spirit never failed to brighten.

What I learned from those times was that the beauty of nature can touch, soothe, and heal our souls at any age. It can provide well-being and satisfaction, no matter what the disability. It became so terribly clear to me: *no senior should be left inside.*

"How lucky you are, Neal, to have this right outside your door."

Neal nods. He expands, though, on my observation. "Yes, but Marcy you can experience this same sense of wonder at a local park or a garden. It's learning to appreciate what you've never been able to see before. Each time I go outside is like going on safari! It's only a different part of the world. Keep your senses on the receiving mode, because like the weather, it's coming at you every day. Admittedly, that's the part you have to work on a little bit – moving from just *looking* to *seeing*. But as you develop this, you will find the world keeps getting bigger, not smaller."

I am hesitant to ask the question I am thinking. But it figures largely in any compass heading on aging. I know Neal's wife of 50 years and partner in much of his work died several years ago. "But what if part of that world – someone you love more than anything – dies?" I decide to delve in.

"There is no fix to that kind of loss," says Neal, truthfully. "When you lose someone like I did, a piece of your world is gone. I guess I'd call what I do now 'quality coping.' I gave up trying to 'move on' or make the pain go away when my wife died. I just incorporate it into living, like losing a leg. You learn to live with that phenomenon rather than trying to fix it. You think about the histories you have, recalling them and reliving them and celebrating the legacy. And while it doesn't take the grief away, it adds more foundation to that mountain you're climbing."

Neal pauses to watch the eagle and osprey swept in a dance in the sky. We both enjoy seeing the osprey cleverly outmaneuver the eagle, who at last gives up the chase and banks away. After the two colorful raptors fade in the distance, Neal puts the binoculars back in his lap. Turning toward me, his expression is thoughtful, as are his next words, which suddenly pull everything together for me. He unveils a stunning view from the destination on the map I am making, and, for a fleeting moment, I am not looking. I can see.

"What is the gift of aging?" he asks. "It is seeking and finding beauty, where many people think beauty isn't. It is taking time to stop, look, and listen.

"The gift of aging is climbing higher and higher up this beautiful mountain that lets you see further and further each day and in every way. The base gets wider and the pinnacle gets higher. And you get to stand on it at no charge, which is the beauty.

"Life experience has built the mountain you stand on. From here, you will find amazing discoveries because you can see far beneath you. The gift is not in answers, no. Instead, the gift is seeing a much bigger view of the questions, which is just as exciting.

"It becomes even more miraculous."

34 THE HEALING POWER OF NATURE

Elizabeth Eckstrom, MD, MPH, MACP

Nature is a healer.

Connection with nature offers physical and mental benefits throughout our life. This is especially true as we age. Older individuals with access to nature – local parks, gardens, green spaces – have improved mental health and cognitive function, fewer physical complaints, and increased social interaction, all of which are key to our well-being.

Society has a problem, though. While our understanding of the health benefits of nature connection continues to grow, we are becoming increasingly *dis*connected from nature. Four out of five Americans, and over half of all people globally, live in urban areas with limited access to natural places. Americans spend more than 90% of their time indoors, and many spend nearly half their day on screens working or consuming media.

Don't be surprised if you hear something new from your doctor: Rather than take a pill, head *outside*. Walk, cycle, garden, sit on a bench in the park. All of these activities are a boon to our bodies and our mental health.

Individuals who are more connected to nature are happier and report more positive life satisfaction. They feel more *vitality*, something I think we all desire as we grow older! But how do natural environments elicit calming responses in us? Exposure to natural settings lowers cognitive "overload" and "mental fatigue." Such restorative environments can ameliorate stress and heighten our coping resources. Access to a park or forest-like area has been shown to correlate with more energy, higher levels of happiness, lower stress, and improved mood and concentration.

What kinds of spaces improve our outlook and overall health? Green ones and blue ones. Green spaces are publicly accessible areas with natural vegetation such as plants, grass, or trees. They include nature reserves, wilderness environments, and urban parks. Blue spaces are beaches, lakes, rivers, and water areas. Backyard gardens are also places to connect with nature. And one extra benefit of growing a garden – either a home, apartment, or community garden – is that you will eat more vegetables! No matter how small the space, bringing nature into your life is important!

In our current culture, many people complain that they are too busy or too tired to make time to get outside every day. Perhaps you are one of them. I hope that naming some *evidence-based health benefits* of nature may help you change your mind! They are:

- reduced stress
- better sleep
- reduced depression
- reduced anxiety
- greater life satisfaction
- increased social connectedness
- lower blood pressure
- improved postoperative recovery
- improved congestive heart failure
- improved pain control
- reduced obesity
- reduced diabetes
- improved immune function
- improved attention
- increased feeling of vigor
- increased longevity

Wow! That is quite an inventory! Let's look a little closer. Research shows that when we walk among woods and trees, we are receiving these hosts of health benefits. First introduced in Japan, *shinrin yoku*, or "forest bathing," is a medical therapy that is now being used worldwide to help improve health and well-being, increase creativity, and fight depression.

Older adults who take daily outdoor walks, runs, or bike rides report more vigor, and fewer complaints about pain, sleep, and other problems, compared to adults who do not go outside daily. People who engage in gardening have better physical functioning, reduced pain, and overall better health status. In terms of mental health, natural environments provide a sense of calm and enhanced mood and facilitate better responses to stressful life events.

Part of the reason for an increase in vitality comes from physical activity associated with nature connection. "Green exercise," as some scientists term it, helps prevent or ameliorate obesity, diabetes, cardiovascular disease, some mental illness, some cancers, and other conditions. Nature connections often also provide social connectedness which is strongly related to good health.

Just one hour spent outdoors in a natural area or garden positively affects an older person's performance of activities of daily living. Overall, people who have more green space in their environments say they feel healthier, no matter what their age. Nearby nature buffers life stresses – a finding demonstrated across all ages and cultures.

People who use the natural environment for physical activity at least once per week have half the risk of poor mental health compared with those who do not do so. Beyond that, each extra weekly activity in nature reduces the risk by a further 6%.

Even *views* of nature have been shown to have positive benefits and be restorative. Residents in care facilities experience increased pleasure if they have a window view where they can observe growing plants, seasonal changes, blooming flowers, and the behavior of birds and other animals. Opportunities for them to "feel nature" are central to life satisfaction. For older adults living in long-term care communities, it is vitally important to provide them opportunities to sit outside in the fresh air, feel the breeze, hear native birds, smell the scents of flowers, even hear rustling leaves – without being separated by glass. This confers well-being, and should be a prime consideration for any kind of residential living.

Nature heals in hospitals, too. Patients have shorter postoperative stays, fewer post-surgical complications, and require less pain medication *if* their windows overlook trees rather than a brick wall.

For vulnerable groups, such as youths at risk, those with mental ill health, and individuals living with dementia, encounters with green spaces are particularly therapeutic. For persons with dementia, being able to engage with the natural world has significant affirmative outcomes, positively influencing eating and sleeping patterns, sense of well-being and esteem, improving social interaction, and a feeling of belonging. Nature connections reduce stress, agitation, anger, and depression.

What happens if an older person is frail and can't get outside by themselves? If at all possible, I recommend that family and friends help them get outside. Assist them to sit in a restful garden area. Or help plant a small garden that will grow flowers and attract birds. If they live in a care facility, take them for drives to places that are meaningful to them. Even just seeing a garden or forest helps with mental restoration, significantly improves mood, reduces the sense of stress, and improves cognitive health. Best of all, sharing outdoor time with children, who also benefit, creates positive intergenerational experiences.

One fascinating new area of research finds that having closeness with nature *throughout one's lifespan* may help people retain an optimistic outlook in old age, even for those with severe health limitations. Having good memories of nature in childhood and middle age provides better coping ability for older people dealing with loss and the stresses and constraints of aging.

Nature connection is restorative throughout our lives, improving physical and mental health, as well as long-term happiness, no matter what our age or situation.

So grab a good jacket, hiking shoes, walking sticks, and *get outside.*

35 THE BEST PLACE IN THE WORLD TO GROW OLD

Elizabeth Eckstrom, MD, MPH, MACP

Want to age well? You might want to move now. The best countries in the world to grow old are ranked by the *Global AgeWatch Index* based on income, employment, health provision, education, and environment. During my research sabbatical, I wanted to see and study these places for myself. That year, Sweden was ranked Number One (since then, Switzerland and Norway have risen to the top. The US loiters much lower: Number 9). I hoped to decipher what lay behind Sweden's status. To do this, I visited public health institutions, hospitals, talked to medical colleagues, and discovered some eye-opening strategies for success.

To begin with, life expectancy in Sweden is among the highest in the world – 79.9 years for men, and 83.7 years for women – second only to Japan; 20% of the Swedish population is over 65 – again, higher than most places in the world. One of the first things I learned was that health has *improved* in the older population over the last few decades, so Sweden's healthcare needs have *decreased* overall.

What is Sweden doing to be such a frontrunner? Immediately, an answer jumps out. Remarkably, Sweden allocates 3.6% of its GDP to long-term care, the home support system for older adults, whereas in the US, the vast majority of long-term care costs are paid by elders and their families. Sweden has the largest healthcare workforce in the world serving citizens over 65. Also, *94% of people over 65 live at home* (wow!), and elders receive in-home assistance when needed.

Sweden has both public and private home-care service programs. Swedes can choose if they want their in-home care covered by public or private funding, so both compete to provide the best care. However, both are funded by the state, *not* by older adults and family. Only 4% of all care – healthcare or home care – is paid for by the patients themselves (how many of us in the US can boast that such a small proportion of our costs is coming out of our pocket?). In addition, much of the care that used to happen in hospitals now happens in the home by healthcare teams.

These provisions alone dramatically increase the well-being of Swedes. There is more, though. Sweden also has numerous home services to try to reduce the impact of the social determinants of health.

One of my favorites is that they have special "municipal fixers" – people who can come in and hang curtains or change lightbulbs and other similar chores to help reduce falls in older adults. That means, if you have been identified as being at high risk for falls, instead of getting out the ladder to change a high lightbulb or clean your gutters, you simply call and have someone come to do it for you – and it is *totally free*.

Swedes do have to apply, and qualify, for these additional benefits. If your needs are high enough, someone can come in every two hours around the clock to help care for you – again, totally without cost to you. Those who receive social services complete a questionnaire once a year rating their satisfaction with the services, and this information is publicly available, so all agencies are incentivized to provide high-quality care.

Sweden also funds programs to train police and other officials in dementia, so they can be part of the solution for struggling families. Dementia awareness is high in Sweden. Every primary care provider is required to ask people 65 and over about their memory at every visit. Sweden has no stigma around dementia, likely helped by the Swedish attitude toward transparency. The Swedish queen is an advocate of this practice because both her parents had dementia. Frequently in the news are tips to prevent Alzheimer Disease and other dementias, and the media makes their coverage positive so people want to follow the guidance.

Older people used to take a lot of drugs – a common fact in many countries – but medication use in Sweden has decreased recently. Every year, the Swedish government develops a list of drugs that older people should not be prescribed, and each clinic has to report how many of these drugs they do prescribe. In addition, there is competition between clinics and counties to have the lowest rates of "bad drug" prescriptions. Even politicians keep track of this and don't want their county to prescribe the most "bad drugs." Swedish primary care providers also have a "Wise List" (drugs that are effective, have few side effects, and are cheaper) and, if they prescribe 90% or more of their drugs from the good list, they get a bonus. Lots of incentives to do the right thing.

Let's go back to the statement I made earlier that Swedish health has improved in the older population over the last few decades, so healthcare needs have decreased overall. Contemplate that for a moment. As healthcare costs continue to skyrocket in the US, how is it that Sweden has actually improved health *and contained costs*?

The answer is pretty straightforward. It is due to all the programs I described, and more. In addition to the incentives to healthcare providers (such as medication prescription programs) to provide top-quality care and services to older adults, Sweden has also implemented *community-based care and practical approaches to older adult safety*, like the "municipal fixers." The country has added many bike lanes to city streets and helps older adults get low-cost bicycles. Falls in the senior population have been greatly reduced by the provision of comprehensive fall prevention programs.

Sweden has implemented multiple creative amenities that are practical, relatively inexpensive, and make a huge difference in quality of life for older adults. When I asked my Swedish colleagues why they had worked so hard and were so determined to truly enhance well-being and health for their older citizens, they simply shrugged their shoulders and replied, "Of course; we couldn't afford to do otherwise."

How Swedish is that?

There are going to be challenges. We can't escape them.
But the question isn't "How can I run away from them?"
What I've learned is, how can I turn this sadness or
frustration or emptiness into something that is positive?

Maggie Vali,
age 79

36 FROM REVOLUTION TO PANDEMIC

Marcy Cottrell Houle

Maggie Vali's effervescent smile never fails to impress me. Now nearing 80, her energy, enthusiasm, and great love of people is legendary among all who know her. Being aware of what she has lived through makes these attributes even more compelling.

"I've always had a positive outlook on life," says Maggie, practically. "No matter how rough things get, I've found there's always a light shining ahead. You just have to have faith, hope, and do the best you can."

An immigrant from Hungary, Maggie makes it sound so easy. I know it's not. I'm familiar with some of her story, and the hardships she's faced: as a girl fleeing her homeland while escaping bullets from machine guns mounted on Russian tanks, living as a refugee in four different countries, losing her beloved husband after 47 years, and surviving breast cancer. Still, Maggie remains uplifted. It makes me want to know more. And I wish to put what I learn from her on the compass dial of my map.

"Tell me again how your mother lost her toes," I ask, only dimly recollecting the harrowing tale.

Maggie chuckles. "Toe. She only lost one. But I'll have to take you back in history a bit to answer that."

She serves me another cup of coffee in her tidy apartment. I've known Maggie for over 40 years, first meeting her at the Bavarian restaurant, Vali's, she and her husband Mike owned for 46 years in the picturesque hamlet of Wallowa Lake.

"My mother lost her toe as a result of the Hungarian Revolution in 1956, but problems in our country began long before that," Maggie begins. "I was born in Transylvania in 1944, which was part of Hungary at the time. For decades, Hungary and Romania had boundary conflicts. Who held the title to Transylvania kept moving back and forth! It was a confusing mess, and mapmakers could barely keep up. For years, our family didn't know if we were Hungarians or Romanians!

"Then, during the Second World War, Germany got involved, as both countries were allies of the Third Reich. At the end of the war, the Soviet Army occupied Hungary and where we lived. The war was over but the mayhem raged on."

"Weren't you frightened?"

"Actually, no. I was surrounded by a large and loving family, and being so young at that time, was virtually unaware of how precarious our situation really was. All I remember is one day when I was 3 I saw my parents quickly packing. They had decided they needed to leave the country, to seek out a better life – *if*, as they explained to me later, we hoped to have a life at all.

"For our family's safety, we left Hungary in 1947. My father was able to book passage on a freighter for the whole family. None of us knew where it was headed. We just got on. And we got off at the first stop: Italy. I had to learn a whole new language!"

Maggie's father, a talented craftsman, stonemason, and sculptor, readily found work. But they didn't stay for long.

"While in Italy, my father heard about the new nation of Israel, opening its doors to refugees and offering them living opportunities. At that time, it wasn't safe to enter Israel because of an ongoing Arab–Israeli war, but my parents decided to head out anyway, and wait near the border. For several months, we lived as refugees in Cairo, Egypt, where my father again found work. Finally, we arrived in Israel in 1948, and, with its open-door policy, were welcomed in."

Once in Israel, the family settled in temporary housing for refugees on a kibbutz, where the whole family could be together, Maggie says. For three years, they lived among people from many countries, all speaking different languages. Maggie enjoyed the vital, polyglot existence. "It was a very pleasant time in our lives. But I had to learn a new language all over again! This time it was Hebrew, which I had to recite in kindergarten! I still can remember some of the fun and lively songs we learned at school," she says with a smile.

After several years, however, Maggie's father began growing homesick for his native land.

"I'm not sure if he knew on some unspoken level that he would not live too much longer. It may have precipitated his desire to return home. But whatever the reason, in 1951, when I was 7, we returned to Hungary anticipating that conditions had improved."

But the situation had not. If anything, circumstances were growing worse. The Soviets were locking down. The family shared a small, two-bedroom apartment in Budapest, near relatives. Then, in 1955, Maggie's father died.

That same year, life in Hungary was visibly changing. Finances were stretched thin for everyone. Food was hard to come by. Under strict Soviet control, life was a continual struggle. There was no freedom of speech, no freedom of press, no freedom of religion or assembly. "Nor was there anyone left you could trust," says Maggie. "Your neighbors, even your family, could turn you in at the slightest suspicion of your not being supportive of the Communist rule."

Yet, at the same time, seeds of revolution were being sown. Writers and journalists began voicing criticism; students started to protest. By 1956, secret activist groups began springing up. Many of those who protested, though, were apprehended and persecuted. It's estimated 2,000 Hungarians were executed and another 100,000 sent to prison."

"People didn't want to entirely overthrow the current government," Maggie explains, "but just to change it to more of a capitalistic government instead of rule by harsh Communist control. Several in my family were protesters. Activists called themselves *The Freedom Fighters*. They hoped to prove to the world that the Hungarian people would not stand for Russian control any longer."

Maggie vividly remembers a day when she was 12 when her uncle came to visit and sounded the alarm.

"My uncle was married to a woman who was a Communist and worked as a secretary; from this, he received a little inside information. He told my mother about rumors he was hearing about serious things happening, and that 'things were going to get worse.'"

Then, on October 23, 1956, the Hungarian uprising began.

"It started with a peaceful demonstration staged by students. The marchers read a list of changes they wanted in the government, including freedom of speech. But during their 'manifesto' a rifle unexpectedly went off. No one knew who was responsible for it, but all suspected it came from the Russian soldiers observing the protest, since no Hungarians were allowed to have a gun."

Chaos immediately broke out. Everyone ran in all directions. Students were arrested and tear gas filled the air. Word got back to Moscow, and within days Russian troops with tanks began pouring into Budapest and spreading across the entire country.

"My uncle came back once more and pleaded with my mother to get out. He told her that he and his wife were planning to escape. He entreated her to think of us – her children. If *we* were to have any chance of survival, we all had to flee immediately."

Maggie's eyes take on a reflective expression as she recalls what happened next.

"Late that night, my mother made the decision to leave everything behind. She and my uncle planned where we would rendezvous. Two days later, on November 8, 1956, we got up before sunrise and dressed in layers, because it was winter and very cold. Just before dawn, we left our home forever. We moved two at a time to avoid suspicion, with instructions to meet up at a designated location a mile away. After that, we all set out on foot together, traveling only at night. It would take seven days of walking to reach the crossing at the Austrian border."

If they were spotted during the day trying to escape, they would have been killed. Making matters more treacherous, they were alerted that mines were planted at the border and weren't sure how to avoid them. By chance, as they neared the crossing, they met a smuggler helping people travel to avoid the explosives.

"Taking all the little money and scant pieces of jewelry we had, he led us safely to a large, open pasture. He pointed in the distance, saying Austria was over there," says Maggie. "He left us with the warning that Russian military trucks, armed with machine guns, continually patrolled the border day and night, using bright, roving spotlights. Tanks passed by every 20 minutes and would shoot to kill anyone who ran."

Maggie well remembers the expansive farm field, dotted with loosely packed haystacks that were considerable in size. The smuggler told the family to hide in these as they made their way across, and to always listen for tanks – you could hear them before seeing them.

"So we moved ever closer to the border, burying ourselves, haystack by haystack, while listening closely for the Russians. At last, we could see the border crossing ahead. A Russian military truck, with rifles gaping and search lights scouring, had just wheeled by. That's when mother yelled to us, *'Run! Run and don't look back!'*"

Maggie ran as she never had before, her life depending on it. She made it to the crossing, and dived into Austria along with her mother, sister, her sister's husband, her brother, and uncle and aunt. They were safe. Her family had made it to freedom.

Maggie's dark brown eyes are bright, even as I can hardly imagine what she endured. "And that's the reason my mother lost her toe! She never complained, poor thing, but suffered terrible frostbite from all the icy cold nights we walked. Much later, in America, a doctor removed the long toe next to her big toe on one foot because it still gave her pain. From then on, she wore a different size shoe on each foot!"

Maggie smiles. I am more familiar with the rest of her story. After her family's escape from Hungary, Maggie and her mother, sister, brother, and brother-in-law were shuttled to a place in Vienna where other refugees lived, all of them uncertain where they would go next. By good fortune, Maggie's family found a sponsor and was selected to go to America for resettlement. In January 1957, soon after Maggie turned 13, they arrived at their new home in Los Angeles.

Once more, Maggie had to learn a new language – this time, English.

"English and Hungarian became my main languages. I forgot most of my Hebrew. And sadly, my Romanian is not all that good.

I lived with my family in California for 16 years, and in 1964, met Mike Vali, who was a friend of my sister's husband. It was love at first sight!"

Maggie was amazed how much they had in common. Mike was a Hungarian refugee. He had been a freedom fighter, and barely escaped Soviet control with his life. "We married in less than a year. Mike didn't like living in congested Los Angeles, so in 1973 we moved to rural northeastern Oregon to start our business. The colder climate was much more like home!"

Their charming alpine delicatessen and restaurant, situated in the shadow of the encircling Wallowa Mountains, thrived under their hard work for four decades. The Valis became an integral part of the community, and had two children. It was during this time that I met Maggie.

In 2005, life for Maggie began to change once more. Mike had a mini-stroke, resulting in physical and memory problems that continued to worsen. Maggie, while caring for him, developed breast cancer. Their son, Mike, and daughter-in-law, Dionne, both trained as chefs, returned home to take over the family legacy. As Mike became increasingly ill, Maggie retired, and they moved to Portland to be closer to their daughter, Monika, a cardiology nurse. She continued to care for Mike and underwent breast cancer treatments. She watched over her husband until he died in 2011.

Maggie is frank about the great loss she felt. "Yes, it was hard, but you can't just close yourself up and wither away. I thought I could handle my sorrow on my own for a time, but my daughter encouraged me to get some help. I joined a support group; we met once a week; there was a lot of tension and heartache, but we tackled our pain and took the bull by the horns. And I found a solution to keep myself from feeling sorry for myself."

"What was that, Maggie?"

"Never give up, and have a better attitude. Go out and take a walk, look at the gorgeous blossoms, the trees, the birds, nature. And the best way to work through your suffering? Helping others. Having compassion for the well-being of others will make you happy. I realized that if I shifted my focus and concern to another person, my own pain lessened."

For a moment I think back to studies I've read by Richard Davidson, a neuroscientist from San Francisco, whose research centers on the theory of a happy brain. It aligns with what Maggie is saying. A positive attitude can indeed influence our sense of well-being. Davidson writes that the fastest way to finding this positivity is to start with love and compassion for others. Our brains feel good when we help others.

There is more to it, though, as I learn from Maggie. What also makes for a positive state, and our happiness, is a sense of gratitude.

"I am grateful just to be alive!" Maggie affirms. "I find joy in waking up every morning. Each day is a gift. You never know if you will have another moment."

I can't help grinning. For as long as I have known her, Maggie has always exuded positivity.

"I learned this, I think, from my mother," Maggie relates. "She had courage and strength and a great outlook on life. Even with all she went through – and she endured many more hardships than I have – she survived and never felt sorry for herself. And perhaps some of my experiences as an immigrant helped shape my perspective."

"In what way?" I ask, curious.

"I think living as a refugee in multiple countries gave me a mindset that helped. It taught me to not be afraid to try new things, even if they might seem scary at first. You can try anything at least once. Have some drive. A go-getter attitude. And if you make a mess of it?" she chuckles, "like I often did with all the languages I had to learn? Well, laugh at yourself! Embrace life!"

If anyone embraces life more than Maggie, I have yet to know them.

"Some of that perspective likely was amplified after my cancer diagnosis," she says. "There were things I used to put too much emphasis on. I don't anymore. They aren't that important. I try to think about what is really worth pursuing. And I don't take anything for granted. It's not that I ignore the negative aspects of life. Instead, I choose to appreciate what is positive."

I latch on to that thought. Positivity is a choice we make.

"There are going to be challenges. We can't escape them. But the question isn't 'How can I run away from them?' What I've learned is, how can I turn this sadness or frustration or emptiness into something that is positive?

"And, as you know, since losing Mike, I am alone. But I'm not lonely. A key is to *surround* yourself with others. I love associating with people of all ages and nationalities and cultures! From little ones to inbetweeners to those who are 95 years old! Because from the oldest ones you can always learn things. Every year, I welcome my age. I'm comfortable with it. I challenge you: look age in the eye! There's no need to be afraid of it. It's just a number, after all. We're all going to get older; we all have aches and pains. But *so what*? Rub something on them, put on the heating pad, and get up and move! I'm just grateful I made it another year. Another day!"

Later that morning, I leave Maggie's apartment – undeniably happier. I plan to return the following month, to ask her a few more questions and to share an authentic Hungarian lunch she has promised to make.

But then something unthinkable happens.

In March 2020, a pandemic, totally unexpected, begins to sweep its cruelty around the world. Like the rest of us in Oregon, Maggie is under quarantine. I call her to see how she is dealing with the scourge of COVID-19, being shut off, isolated, and living all alone. For many seniors, the terrible virus hits them the hardest, with the most dire consequences.

I should have known before even dialing her number that Maggie would offer a different assessment on the pandemic. That she could somehow shine a positive light on a calamitous situation. It is something I long to hear right now. When she answers the phone, Maggie's voice is unchanged. It is unafraid, calm, even affirmative.

"It's easy to think this is the worst thing that has ever happened. And it is a tragedy. But people who lived through history know something different. This is not the end; this isn't hopeless. And some things in life might turn out better than they were before."

It is not Maggie's attitude that surprises me but her opinion that some elements might be improved. "What things, Maggie?"

"Life in Hungary, before the revolution, might offer some lessons for living now," she says. "In the old days, people took more time to be together. They cooked together, played together, spent more time together as a family. But in modern times – and I've seen this even with my own family – we don't have time for that because our lives are too busy.

"And another difference – a big difference from the old times: young people don't pay much attention to old people anymore. Yet what they would learn if they would stop and listen to some of them! And old timers would relish it because we love to reminisce and remember things and share them," she chuckles. "But a lot of grandkids now don't have the time or tendency to listen and are impatient. They say, 'What do you know? You're *old*.' I was never raised that way."

"How was it different then, growing up in Hungary?"

"We always had respect for older people, and especially our grandparents," she replies. "If you were riding on a bus and saw an older person standing, you'd get up and give them your seat. If you saw someone older carrying groceries, you would cross the street and help them without even asking. And it didn't even have to be a person who was "old"; it could be someone only five years older than you! Even an older sibling! It was just drilled into us: *Respect for others.* That was our culture, how we were raised. We took care of our parents and grandparents as they got older."

Her tone becomes more buoyant. "But perhaps we will all learn something from this pandemic. Maybe we will develop a renewed appreciation for each other and for the great gift it is to spend time together. Maybe it's a sign that we need to love one another, respect our elders. Most of all, to be kind to each other."

A vision of a kinder world, right now, seems far away. But perhaps Maggie is right. It is an attitude to hold on to.

She asks about my family and after telling me about hers assures me she is doing just fine. "I think the hard experiences

I have lived through help, and have made me a stronger person,"
she reflects. "Through them I learned to value life and people –
whoever they are, wherever they come from. They helped me to
see that *the path to joy is that of connection.* And even though we're
forced to be isolated right now, we can still reach out. So, after
talking to me, get back on the phone! Skype! Write a letter or send
a card!"

I can only imagine how many cards Maggie has written, how
many friends she has touched.

"The idea is that you are thinking of someone else," Maggie
says. "It doesn't take a lot of effort to write a note, but it will bring
someone joy, just as it brings *you* joy to sit down and think about
that person." She pauses for a moment, then says thoughtfully,
"Facing this pandemic is a little like hiding in haystacks."

"What do you mean?"

"We're concealing ourselves from the enemy, but we know we
are in this *together.* We will get through this, and, even though this
is different from anything I've experienced, some things are the
same. If we all do what we're supposed to do, keep our faith and
have courage, and recognize the need we have for one another,
then we'll be fine."

Somehow the terrifying virulence of the pandemic has just been
dealt a swift blow.

And while I can't see Maggie as she shares her words, I know
just what her youthful, lively, elfin face looks like.

Her dark brown eyes are sparkling. And, as always, she is
smiling.

37 THE POWER OF POSITIVITY

Elizabeth Eckstrom, MD, MPH, MACP

Maggie Vali has a lot to teach us. Enduring turmoil most of us in the United States will not know, she never fails to thrive. How is this possible? Maggie answers that question simply, "I've always had a positive outlook on life. No matter how rough things get, I've found there's always a light shining ahead. You just have to have faith, hope, and do the best you can."

Positivity. This one attribute can predict one's ability to bounce back from life's inevitable stresses. Taking time to learn skills to self-generate positive emotions will help us become healthier, more resilient, and more connected to others and the world around us.

How we think about things influences our health, well-being, happiness, and effectiveness more than outward circumstances themselves. Life can be full of joy and satisfaction even amidst difficulty and obstacles. Maggie is clear: nothing is hopeless. Psychiatrist Dr. Karl Menninger professed, "Attitudes are more important than facts."

But positive emotions do more than make us "feel happy." Current research suggests strong links between our outlook and our health. There is a strong mind/body connection. What happens in our thinking influences what happens in our body. Possessing greater optimism can lower the risk of developing chronic diseases.

Dr. Alan Rozanski, cardiologist at Mount Sinai in New York, in his studies of positivity, found that people who ranked high in optimism were significantly less likely to have a heart attack, and had lower mortality rates from any cause, than did pessimists. In a meta-analysis published in the *Journal of the American Medical*

Association that looked at 15 studies measuring optimism and pessimism with pooled data of 209,436 individuals, people with the most optimistic outlook had a 35% lower risk for cardiovascular events.

Pessimism increases inflammation in the body. It more readily activates a "fight or flight" response in our system, which over time can wear our bodies down.

In contrast, cultivating positivity can boost our immune system. Developing a positive attitude can help lower blood pressure and maintain healthy blood sugar levels. Those who have positive outlooks have greater odds of achieving "exceptional longevity." Independent of one's socioeconomic status, health conditions, smoking, diet, and alcohol use, optimism is a critical psychosocial resource for extending lifespan in older adults.

Optimists have the ability to reframe challenging circumstances by their attitudes toward them. They react to life's trials in less stressful ways. Even those in poor health or with poor prognoses can moderate and recast their health outcomes by their attitudes.

Ann Crumpacker, at age 94, and with multiple health conditions, exemplifies this well. On a day Marcy and I went to visit her at her apartment, we asked what her secret to keeping such a positive attitude was in the face of her medical challenges. Ann was swift in her response.

"I have never been one to feel sorry for myself. When someone says, 'It's not fair,' I would say back to them, 'Well, now who ever told you it would be?'" She pointed to a note written in calligraphy and framed on her desk. "It's my motto," she told us with a smile. *"Don't stew; do."*

Understandably, people wonder: Isn't your attitude predetermined? If you view life as half-empty, won't you always feel that way? Thankfully, as we learned from Dan Buettner and others who study happiness, 40% of our happiness is under our control. Buettner suggests the following ways to optimize happiness: pick a job you love over money, socialize in person seven hours a day, try new things, have sexual intercourse twice per week, sleep seven hours a night, own a dog, be in love, have kids, and live in the right place. In the US, the happiest communities are bikeable, have good food, and city government focuses on civic life.

Admittedly, it's not always easy to have a positive attitude, especially if life doesn't seem to turn out the way you want it to. In fact, for many people, positive thinking seems "too simplistic," "too unrealistic," just a fool's "pipe dream," and contrary to their nature. Yet the benefits of developing a positive attitude cannot be overstated. Having a can-do attitude helps us persist in overcoming life's obstacles rather than giving up and thinking there's nothing we can do about a bad situation.

Judith Moskowitz, Ph.D., MPH, Director of Research at Northwestern Medicine's Osher Center for Integrative Medicine, concludes that positive emotions are uniquely beneficial in relation to longevity, better health, and better psychological well-being. Through her research, she developed eight skills that can help foster positive emotions. If we practice some or all of them, they can help us better cope with stress and find contentment in our lives.

1   Recognize a positive event each day (it can be as small as a good cup of coffee!).
2   Savor that event. Write it down in a journal.
3   Take time to feel grateful for something like your family or a friend. Start a daily gratitude journal.
4   Practice mindfulness. Be aware of your thoughts. When a negative musing pops into your head, quickly substitute it with something else – a scripture, a better thought.
5   Reframe events and your appraisal of them.
6   Recognize your personal strengths. Recall them. Are you a good friend? Are you kind? Can you make people laugh? Remember you have personal skills.
7   Work toward attainable goals. When people set realistic goals and make progress toward them, they feel positive emotions and a sense of accomplishment.
8   Practice acts of kindness.

This last suggestion is especially powerful. Acts of kindness make us feel better and healthier. They can be as simple as opening a door for someone, or giving a person a smile. People who are kind to others are happier and feel more connected to the world.

And in terms of aging well, our attitude can make all the difference. How we respond to aging is more than circumstances; *it is a choice we can make in our minds.* We have seen how banishing ageism from our thinking and having a positive outlook on our own aging can add 7.5 years to our lives. Research shows having faith and a strong spiritual life can amplify our longevity and happiness.

Turning our thoughts outward rather than inward, reducing the self-focus of our vision, cultivating compassion for others, ultimately is a pathway to developing a positive attitude toward life. The result?

As Rabbi Josh Stampfer says, "when you care about the welfare of others more than yourself, when you wipe the tears from the eyes of another, you will discover *joy.*"

38 AN INCREDIBLE JOURNEY

Marcy Cottrell Houle

The map is nearly done. There is only one thing more to add.

From where I am now standing, just for a moment, I can see the summit. A rare break in the fog swirling below the crown of the mountain allows me to see that there's still more of the trail ahead. There are boulders to scramble and paths leading to false summits. Yet the view leaves me with something unshakable.

This trail is one I *want* to take to its final climb. For from this vantage point, I have seen its beauty.

An accident got me started on this journey. Who in their right mind thanks an accident for changing a life course? Yet it made me face my trepidations and step out on a path most of us dread to think about. Like many, I feared growing old.

Then, I started walking.

I carried a compass but had no map. To make one, I began asking questions. I sought explanations from Elizabeth to provide bearings for my heading. From Wendy, I became aware of why I needed to plan. Those who were farther ahead of me on the trail provided surveillance on what lay ahead.

Soon, I began making discoveries I never knew, about aging. Those who did it well spoke of real joy. They looked at things in new ways, going deeper, and finding greater meaning. They shared, even amidst sorrow, a love of life.

From them all, I learned lessons. Preparation for the trip is vital. Realize the passage will take effort. Developing mindfulness is key. Always stay attentive to surroundings, because there are ghost trails setting off in dangerous directions. Some contours I can go around but others I must cross over. When the storm clouds appear – and they will – keep a positive spirit and an attitude of hope.

Along the entire journey, it is paramount to have a sense of purpose. Make these years count. Maintain a compassionate concern for future generations, and seek to do something good for them and for our earth. Feel gratitude for life. As much as possible, try to remain close to nature. Nature brings happiness. And always – always – treasure family and friends.

At the same time, expect some segments of the journey will be difficult, sad, and discouraging. There will be loss. But even then, these guides tell me, there are rewards all along the way.

Looking at my map now, I see it is flecked with sparkling gifts I could never have imagined.

There is one more wayfinder, though, I need to mark. I realize it's been there all along, but it grows in prominence as I get closer to making the climb. Lucille Pierce, the calligrapher who will be 102 this year, puts it into words – words that I will place on my final map and engrave upon this cairn.

"Each phase of life has its blessings, as well as its trials, so enjoy what you can now. And as far as I know, this is the only chance we get. Old age isn't so frightening. Do all that you can to stay healthy, keep active both mentally and physically, then recognize that all things eventually wear out and you will too. It helps to be able to laugh at yourself! Remember, death itself is just another phase of life.

"I've been lucky. I've enjoyed a long-lasting faith that provides a supportive community and guide. I'm not sure what follows this precious life on earth, but my faith gives me, not fear, but a grand sense of wonder about it. In life and death, we have only to do one thing:

Simply, let Love in."

AFTERWORD

Elizabeth Eckstrom, MD, MPH, MACP

At 100 years old, Captain Tom Moore, a decorated British Army officer from World War II, walked 100 laps of an 82-foot walk on the brick patio next to his garden and raised £32.8 million, or $40 million, for the National Health Service to treat COVID-19. At 78 years old, Joseph Biden, Jr., assumed the office of the presidency of the United States. Before her death at 87 years old, US Supreme Court Justice Ruth Bader Ginsburg continued to impact important policy decisions in the United States which also affect the entire world.

In some people's view, these people may be "old." But their contributions to society have no age.

The people Marcy has interviewed and the stories we have told in this book show us that growing old may not be easy, but it can be incredibly rewarding and meaningful. Embracing **positivity, planning, and perseverance** can help ensure we thrive into our 80s, 90s, 100s.

Today, the average *lifespan* in the United States approaches 80 years old. However, the average *healthspan* – the number of healthy years we live – is much shorter in the US, at 63 years old. This means we are living much longer than we are healthy. Further, the disparity in healthspan is substantial in this country. Those most privileged have a healthspan that approaches their lifespan.

If we are to succeed in the future, we must ensure that everyone has the opportunity to match their healthspan to their lifespan. In this book, I have tried to document ways to improve and augment health and life satisfaction, and to answer questions we didn't address in our first book – helping your brain thrive, how to optimize your independence – as well as to offer realistic guideposts on what to expect with normal aging.

We hope this front-line information will enable our readers to set their own compass, chart their own path, and overcome obstacles that appear along the way. Creating a positive frame-work for aging – one where healthspan can match lifespan – allows you, and the community of people you impact, the oppor-tunity to succeed as well as those whose stories we have told in this book, and live with creativity, vitality, activity, and purpose.

"The Elders" is an organization started by Nelson Mandela. Its members have included Jimmy Carter, Kofi Anon, Desmond Tutu, Mary Robinson, and many others. Its vision is of a world where "people live in peace, conscious of their common humanity and their shared responsibilities for each other, for the planet and for future generations" (www.theelders.org). In traditional society, as we have learned from David Barrios, elders always had a role in conflict resolution, long-term decision making, and applying wis-dom where it was needed. We need these global elders. They create unified action to help resolve the world's most intractable chal-lenges. They help us understand that it is crucial to put aging well at the center of policy internationally to harness the power of older people and move forward globally. "Walk together, work together, learn together, speak out together, change the world together."

I hope we can all become elders who have this kind of impact on our world.

It *is* possible.

ACKNOWLEDGMENTS

We would like to acknowledge Dr. Emily Morgan, Assistant Professor at Oregon Health & Science University, for her contributions to Chapter 12, "Brain Health across the Lifespan: What Can I Do NOW to Prevent Dementia Later On?" I first appreciated the concept of "last in, first out" when Dr. Morgan gave multiple talks on this topic several years ago, and it has really helped me frame how I think about healthy brain aging. The "Brain Health across the Lifespan" chapter closely aligns with Dr. Morgan's work. We would also like to acknowledge Dr. Gracey McGrory, an Emergency Medicine resident at the University of Nevada, Las Vegas. Dr. McGrory helped with background research for Part II of the book while she was a medical student at Oregon Health & Science University. We are so grateful for both their valuable contributions.

We are so appreciative of the informative chapters written by Wendy K. Goidel, Esq., founding and managing member of the Goidel Law Group PLLC and its Estate Planning and Elder Law Center. Wendy's passion for elders and her tireless work to improve their quality of life are showcased in this book and give us a critical planning piece that can help us all age well.

We also wish to thank Darla Philips, PT, DPT, ATC, OCS – an extraordinary physical therapist in Portland, Oregon, who has helped countless patients deal with pain issues that many providers had previously given up on. Her chapter on pain relief offers a tremendous measure of hope, regardless of our age.

Our deepest appreciation goes to all of the elders who gave their time to share personal stories and thoughts: David Barrios; Lilly Cohen; Neal Maine; Bob Moore; Lucille Pierce; Barbara Roberts and Don Nelson; Eleanore Rubenstein; Rabbi Joshua Stampfer; Susan Tolle, telling the story of her mother, Mary Hughes; Maggie

Vali; and Karen Wells. The wisdom they shared provided a unique dimension to this book that could be found nowhere else. Each was a true inspiration to both of us. We cherish the friendships that have developed with them, which mean so much to us.

Lastly, we want to thank our families for their resolute support and love. Traveling the trails together with them makes the aging journey one of joy!

Appendix: Elizabeth's Original Mediterranean Diet Recipes

Farro, Arugula, and Tomato Salad

I had a salad similar to this on a beautiful spring afternoon while in Trevi, Italy.

Ingredients
- 1 cup (128 g) farro (also called spelt)
- 2 cups (256 g) cherry tomatoes, halved
- 2 cups (256 g) baby arugula
- Good olive oil
- 2 cloves garlic, minced
- A pinch of dried red chili flakes
- 2 cups (475 ml) water

"Toast" the farro, garlic, and red chili flakes for 6–8 minutes on medium to low heat (or until the farro turns light brown and the mixture is fragrant) on the stove top in a large frying pan, with a generous amount of olive oil. Then, add 2 cups of water and simmer till all the water is absorbed (this could take 15–45 minutes, depending on your farro). If the farro is still too chewy, add extra water. Cool the ingredients completely, and then add the tomatoes, arugula, and some good sea salt. Add a little more olive oil if needed. Serve and enjoy!

Delicata Squash and Mushroom Salad

Serves 2 for a generous dinner portion.

Ingredients

- 1 medium sized delicata squash
- 1 medium shallot, sliced thin
- 2 cups (256 g) shitake mushrooms, sliced thin
- 2–3 cups (~300 g) fresh spinach
- ¼ cup (32 g) walnuts, toasted

Cut delicata squash in half length-wise. Remove seeds. Slice crosswise into ¼–⅓-inch slices. Spread in a single layer on a baking sheet. Spread shallots evenly over the squash. Bake at 400 °F for 25 minutes, or until lightly browned and soft but not mushy. Turn squash half-way through cooking so both sides get some nice browning.

While squash is cooking, slice the mushrooms and sauté in a little olive oil. Toast the walnuts.

As squash and mushrooms are finishing, start the dressing (you want everything to be hot at once).

Dressing

- 1 tsp (5 g) dried porcini mushrooms, soaked in a very small amount of water (just enough to soften them) for 20 minutes and minced fine (start soaking them before you put the squash in the oven)
- 2–3 cloves garlic, minced
- 1 tbsp (15 g) fresh sage leaves, minced
- Olive oil
- Splash Balsamic vinegar

Put minced porcini, garlic, sage into olive oil in a small skillet. Sauté just till garlic starts to brown and sage releases its fragrance – 2–3 minutes. Turn heat off, add balsamic, and season with salt and pepper.

Place spinach in bowls. Cover with squash/shallots, then mushrooms, then dressing, then walnuts. Stir gently, then serve hot.

Brussels Sprout Salad

Serves 2.

Ingredients

- 1 lb Brussels sprouts. Get small to medium Brussels sprouts as they will be the right size and taste the best.
- Olive oil spray
- Spinach
- 1 medium shallot
- Olive oil, about 2–3 tbsp (30–45 ml)
- Splash balsamic vinegar
- Herbes de Provence
- Shaved asiago (use a carrot peeler)

Halve Brussels sprouts and score the core so they cook evenly. Place cut side down on a cookie sheet that has been sprayed with olive oil spray. Spray the tops of the Brussels sprouts with olive oil. Roast at 375 °F for about 20–25 minutes, until softened but not mushy. You may need to flip them after 15–20 minutes, but not always.

While Brussels sprouts are roasting, slice shallot very thin. Place in a small frying pan with olive oil, Herbes de Provence, and a little salt and pepper. Cook over medium heat till the shallot is caramelized (lightly brown and a little crispy). Remove from heat, add a few drops of balsamic vinegar, and immediately pour over the spinach to wilt it.

Add the roasted Brussels sprouts to the already dressed spinach. Top with shaved asiago and serve immediately.

Citrus and Avocado Salad

This salad is great during the winter when citrus and avocados are good. Serves 2.

Ingredients

- 1 orange, peeled and quartered then sliced

(cont.)

- 1 grapefruit, each section individually peeled (this goes pretty fast after you figure out how to do it – but you can also skip this ingredient and use 2 oranges instead)
- ¼ cup (32 g) slivered almonds, toasted
- 1 avocado, chopped into about 1 cm chunks just before serving
- Spinach

Dressing
- 2–3 tbsp (30–45 ml) grapeseed oil
- ½ tbsp (8 g) sugar
- 1 tbsp (15 g) zested orange rind (remember to do this before you peel the orange!)
- 1 tbsp (15 g) finely minced shallot
- 1 tbsp (15 ml) champagne citrus vinegar
- 1 tbsp (25 ml) lemon juice
- Pinch salt
- Sprinkle pepper

Prep oranges, grapefruit, and toasted almonds.

Make dressing.

Assemble salad – place spinach in bottom of bowl, then citrus, avocado. Dress liberally. Sprinkle toasted almonds on top. I like to serve it in individual bowls to be mixed well by guests before eating.

Grilled Zucchini and Red Pepper Salad

Serves 2.

Ingredients
- 1 medium zucchini
- ¼ cup (32 g) pine nuts

(cont.)

- Cut 1 red pepper into small pieces
- Crumble ~⅓ cup (43 g) feta - I like sheep's-milk feta

Dressing

- 2–3 tbsp (30–45 ml) olive oil
- 1 tsp (5 ml) balsamic vinegar
- pinch Herbes de Provence
- salt, pepper
- 1–2 cloves garlic

Toast the pine nuts. Put lots of spinach, pine nuts, red pepper, feta into bowl. Make the dressing.

Cut zucchini in half lengthways and spray with olive oil spray, then sprinkle with Herbes de Provence.

Now that you have everything prepped, turn on your grill.

Grill zucchini about 3–4 minutes per side, till softened and with good grill marks but not mushy.

Take the zucchini off the grill and quickly slice them up. Put on salad and toss quickly to mix. Dress the salad and mix again. Serve immediately.

Grilled Zucchini, Tomato, Basil, and Fresh Mozzarella Salad

This update to the classic salad will have you hooked the first time you try it! An Elizabeth original. Don't make this if you don't have garden tomatoes.

Serves 2–3, depending on the size of your zucchinis.

- Slice 2 medium-sized zucchinis in ⅓–½-inch (2–2.5-cm) slices the long way (for ease of grilling). Spray both sides with olive oil spray, and sprinkle one side with Herbes de Provence, salt, and pepper.

(cont.)

- Slice 2–3 large garden tomatoes about the same thickness as the zucchini.
- Slice 1 8 oz (240 g) ball of fresh mozzarella into very thin slices. Make sure you have enough tomatoes and mozzarella to completely cover the zucchini.
- Sliver about 12 leaves of garden basil into thin strips.

Grill zucchini on medium hot grill till they have nice grill marks, flip, and repeat on other side. They should be soft but not mushy. Watch them constantly so as not to overcook. Total time on the grill about 3–4 minutes per side.

Spread grilled zucchini in a single layer on a big platter. Immediately place the sliced mozzarella on the hot zucchini (so it will get all soft and melty). Top with a layer of sliced tomatoes. Spread the basil on top and then drizzle with your best olive oil and sprinkle with fleur de sel. Serve immediately.

Salmon Cooked in Parchment Paper with Dry Rub

Heat oven to 400.
- De-bone ~1.25–1.5 lb (500–700 g) salmon or steelhead fillet

Mix Rub (proportions are approximate, adjust for your own taste):
- ½ tbsp (7.5 g) paprika
- ½ tbsp (7.5 g) chili powder
- 1 tsp (5 g) garlic salt
- 1 tsp cumin (5 g)
- ½ tsp salt (2.5 g)
- ½ tsp ginger (2.5 g)
- ¼ tsp dry mustard (1.25 g)
- 1½ tbsp (22 g) brown sugar

(cont.)

Pat rub on top of salmon fillet – should be pretty thick. Wrap in parchment paper and cook 12–17 minutes (depending on size and thickness of salmon fillet). Remove from oven and let sit another 5 minutes before opening the parchment paper. Serve immediately with roasted asparagus or sautéed spinach with garlic.

Tuna, Delicata Squash, and Sautéed Spinach

This is a fantastic dinner combination! Serves 2.

Ingredients

- 1 delicata squash
- I medium shallot, sliced into thin slices
- ½ lb (225 g) sushi grade ahi steak
- Olive oil
- Olive oil spray
- 6–8 cups spinach
- pinch dried red chili flakes
- 3 cloves minced garlic
- few drops of sesame oil
- 1 tsp (5 g) sesame seeds
- 1–2 tsp (5–10 ml) soy sauce plus more for tuna
- Wasabi to taste

Squash: Cut 1 delicata squash in half length-wise. Remove seeds. Slice crosswise into ¼–⅓-inch (~ 0.75 cm) slices. Spread in a single layer on a baking sheet.

Spread thinly sliced shallots evenly over the squash.

Bake at 400 °F for 25 minutes, or until lightly browned and soft, but not mushy. Turn squash half-way through cooking so both sides get some nice browning.

(cont.)

Tuna: get ½ lb (225 g) sushi grade ahi steak. Spray or brush a thin layer of olive oil on both sides. Lightly season with salt and pepper. Let sit for a few minutes.

Prepare spinach: place small amount olive oil, pinch dried red chili flakes, 3 cloves garlic, a few drops of sesame oil, 1 tsp (5 g) sesame seeds, and 1–2 tsp (5–10 ml) soy sauce in a wok.

When the squash is about 10 minutes from done, turn on the wok. Cook a few minutes until garlic just starts to brown. Add lots and lots of spinach and stir till it is wilted.

When squash and spinach are just about done, put the tuna on a grill that has been heated to 550 °F. Cook one minute on each side for a rare sear.

Arrange squash, tuna, and spinach on plates. Serve wasabi and soy sauce on the side for the tuna.

INDEX